THE SIRTFOOD DIET

The complete beginner's guide to lose weight and transform your body, burn fat, activate your metabolism and get lean. Include a 7-day meal plan and recipes.

Ava J. Li

Text Copyright © Ava J. Li

All rights reserved. No part of this guide may be reproduced in any form without permission in writing from the publisher except in the case of brief quotations embodied in critical articles or reviews.

Legal & Disclaimer

The information contained in this book and its contents is not designed to replace or take the place of any form of medical or professional advice; and is not meant to replace the need for independent medical, financial, legal or other professional advice or services, as may be required. The content and information in this book has been provided for educational and entertainment purposes only.

The content and information contained in this book has been compiled from sources deemed reliable, and it is accurate to the best of the Author's knowledge, information and belief. However, the Author cannot guarantee its accuracy and validity and cannot be held liable for any errors and/or omissions. Further, changes are periodically made to this book as and when needed. Where appropriate and/or necessary, you must consult a professional (including but not limited to your doctor, attorney, financial advisor or such other professional advisor) before using any of the suggested remedies, techniques, or information in this book.

Upon using the contents and information contained in this book, you agree to hold harmless the Author from and against any damages, costs, and expenses, including any legal fees potentially resulting from the application of any of the information provided by this book. This disclaimer applies to any loss, damages or injury caused by the use and application, whether directly or indirectly, of any advice or information presented, whether for breach of contract, tort, negligence, personal injury, criminal intent, or under any other cause of action.

You agree to accept all risks of using the information presented inside this book.

You agree that by continuing to read this book, where appropriate and/or necessary, you shall consult a professional (including but not limited to your doctor, attorney, or financial advisor or such other advisor as needed) before using any of the suggested remedies, techniques, or information in this book.

Table of Contents

It's true that 6 out of every 10 Americans are currently struggling to live their lives through the pain and discomfort of disease, but these statistics don't have to keep declining. You now have enough knowledge to make lifestyle changes that are going to protect you from being on the wrong end of these statistics.

There are too many diseases and medical conditions caused by the food we eat. The quality of food has decreased dramatically over the past decades as the food-processing industry is now providing most of the food we consume.

The more processed the food type is, the more harmful it is to your body. Food-processing companies are providing poison for the consumers, just to make more profits.

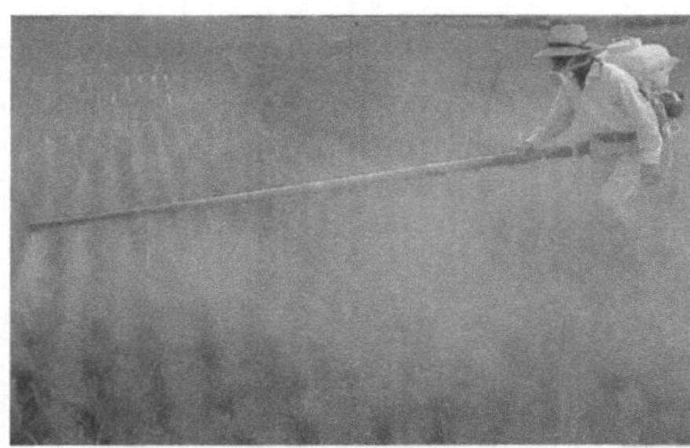

It is very difficult to find organic food nowadays as farmers use different chemicals to grow crops, fruits, and vegetables while animals are fed with concentrated food to grow very fast before being slaughtered for meat. All these chemicals are affecting the quality of food and our health.

There is way too much processed food introduced to us, and the Western way of life encourages the consumption of junk food. This is the main reason why diabetes and obesity are becoming very common in Western countries, especially in the United States.

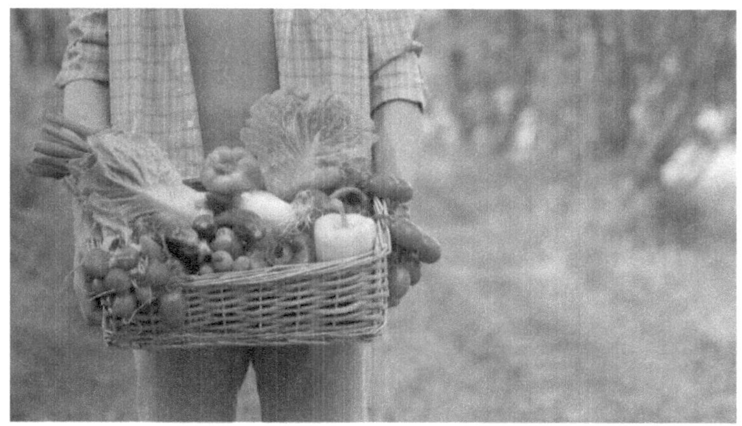

This processed-food madness should now stop, and the sirtfood diet is here to do so. This meal plan developed in the UK is trying to create a strong reputation in the United States. The logic behind this diet is very interesting, as it has a different approach to food than other diets.

If you are struggling with your weight, don't have too much energy, and also have the suspicion of having different diseases caused by bad nutrition, then this is the diet for you.

Don't hesitate and try the sirtfood diet now!

Enjoy reading!

Chapter 1
What is a sirtfood diet

The sirtfood diet is a diet named after a molecule in some plant-based foods, called sirtuin activators.

Sirtuin activators are a type of protein that helps insulate cells from the effect of ageing, inflammation and several nasty metabolic processes.

Owing to this, sirtuin activators have been associated with longevity, with people who intake high amounts of sirtuin over long periods demonstrably living longer than their peers. There are also numerous other benefits, such as increases in muscle mass and making it easier to burn. The sirtfood diet revolves around, ensuring you keep your sirtuin intake high, promoting weight loss and overall bodily health.

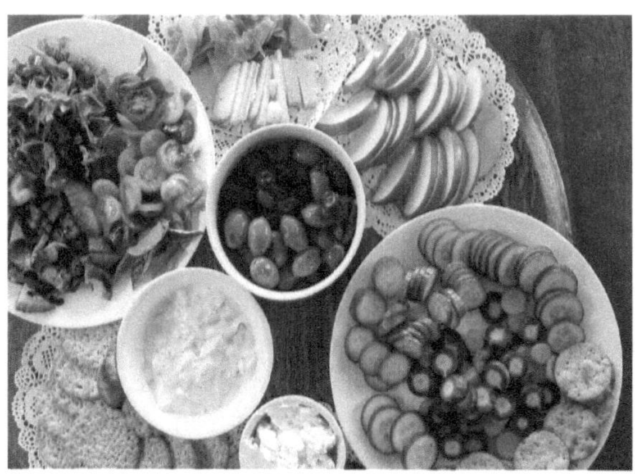

The interesting part of the sirtfood diet is its shift in focus. This isn't a fad diet to lose weight rather the emphasis is just eating in a healthy and balanced way, with weight loss naturally occurring once your body has been cleansed of your poor eating habits.

There are many foods which contain sirtuin activators, most notably both chocolate and red wine. Of course, the sirtuin diet doesn't claim to be a miracle diet where you can binge on chocolate and wine, if only hey!. You will still need to balance your intake of calories and ensure you receive an even spread of essential food groups too.

The core of the diet consists of healthy sirtuin activator foods, which includes blueberries, apples, strawberries, soy, olive oil, green tea, turmeric, citrus fruits, red onion and kale. There are also a couple of surprises, such as coffee, which is usually reprimanded in most contemporary diets.

However, the problem with fasting diets, as the name implies, is that you have to fast. Fasting feels awful, especially when we are surrounded by other people having regular eating habits. It also puts some social spotlight on your own diet – explaining to your co-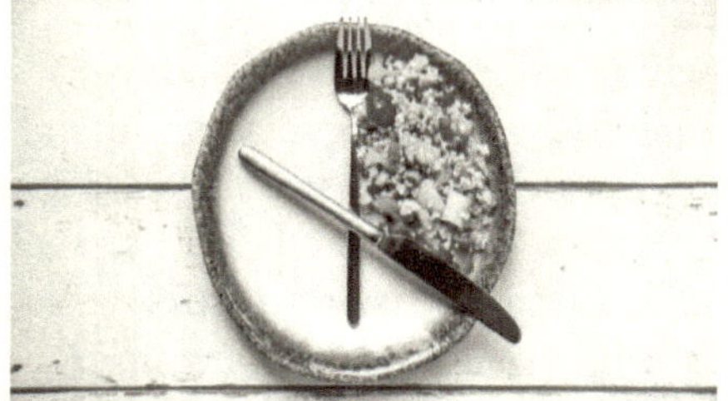workers or your extended family why you are not eating on certain days is bound to generate incredulity and challenges to your diet regime. Furthermore, even though fasting has numerous associated benefits, there are some downsides too. Fasting is associated with muscle loss, as the body doesn't discriminate between muscle mass and fat tissue when choosing cells to burn for energy.

Fasting also risks malnutrition, simply by not eating enough foods to get essential nutrients. This risk can be somewhat alleviated by taking vitamin supplements and eating nutrient-rich foods, but fasting can also slow and halt the digestive system altogether preventing the absorption of supplements. These supplements also need dietary fat to be dissolved, which you might also lack if you were to implement a strict fasting.

On top of this, fasting isn't appropriate for a huge range of people. Obviously, you don't want children to fast and potentially inhibit their growth. Likewise, the elderly, the ill and the pregnant are all just too vulnerable to the risks of fasting.

Additionally, there are several psychological detriments to fasting, despite commonly being associated with spiritual revelations. Fasting makes you irritable and causes you to feel slightly on edge your body is telling you constantly that you need to forage for food, enacting physical processes that affect your mood and emotions.

This is why the authors of the sirtfood diet sought a replacement for fasting diets. Fasting is beneficial for our body, but it just isn't practical for society at large. This is where sirtuin activators and sirtfoods come to the rescue.

Sirtuins were first discovered in 1984 in yeast molecules. Of course, once it became apparent that sirtuin activators affected a variety of factors, such as lifespan and metabolic activity, interest in these proteins blossomed.

Sirtuin activators boost your mitochondria's activity, the part of the biological cell which is responsible for the production of energy. This, in turn, mirrors the energy-boosting effects, which also occur due to exercise and fasting. The sirtfood diet is thought to start a process called adipogenesis, which prevents fat cells from duplicating which should interest any potential dieter.

The interesting part is that the sirtuin activators influence your genetics. The notion of the 'genetic' lottery is embedded in the public consciousness, but genes are more changeable then you might think. You won't be able to change your eye color or your height, but you can activate or deactivate specific genes based on environmental factors. This is called epigenetics, and it is a fascinating field of study.

Sirtuin activators cause the sir genes to activate, the before-mentioned 'skinny genes', which in turn increases the release of sirts. Sirts or silent information regulators also help regulate the circadian rhythm, which is your natural body clock and influences sleep patterns.

Sleep is important for many vital biological processes, including those that help regulate blood sugar (which is also important for losing weight). If you find yourself constantly stuck in a state of lag and brain fog, this may be caused by your circadian rhythm being out of sync, which is another way the sirtfood diet can help your body.

Additionally, sirts help contain free radicals. Free radicals are not as awesome as the sound they are particles in your body that damage your DNA and speed up the ageing process.

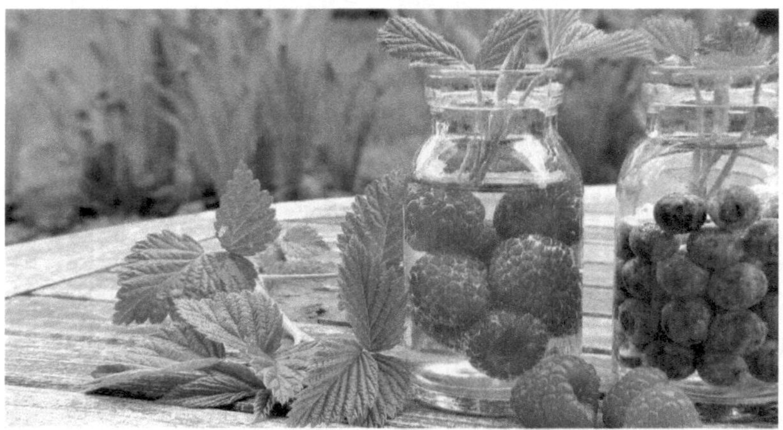

To summarize, the sirtfood diet contains foods which are high in sirtuin activators. Sirtuin activators activate your sir genes or 'skinny genes' which enact beneficial metabolic processes. These processes, which involve molecules, called sirts, causes your body to burn fat, repair bodily cells and combat free radicals.

So, sirtfoods have been hailed as the next dietary wonder but where is the cold, hard evidence? Well, the evidence for the sirtfood diet comes from multiple sources. To start with, Aidan Goggins and Glen Matten, the originators of the sirtfood diet, performed their own trial at a privately owned fitness center to test sirtfoods themselves.

At a fitness center in Chelsea, London, the two authors of the sirtfood diet made a selection of their clientele eat a carefully monitored constructed sirtfood diet. What is particularly interesting about the study is that weight wasn't the only variable measured the researchers also measured body composition and metabolic activity they were searching for the holistic effect of the diet.

97.5% of people managed to stick to the first-three day fasting period, involving only 1,000 calories. Generally speaking, this is a much higher rate of success than typical fasting diets, where many people have their willpower shattered in just the first few days.

Out of the 40 participants, 39 completed the study. In terms of overall fitness and weight, the individuals in the study were well distributed 2 were officially obese, 15 fell into the overweight category while 22 had a regular body mass index. There were also 21 women and 18 men a diet for both the genders! However, with that being said, being members of a fitness center, the individuals in the study were more likely to exercise more than the standard population a potential confounding factor.

Participants lost over 7lbs on average in the first week. Every participant experienced an improvement in body composition, even if their gains were not as dramatic as their peers.

There were also numerous reported psychological benefits, although these were not formally quantified. These improvements include an overall sense of feeling and looking better. As a side note, it was also claimed the 40 participants rarely felt hungry, even despite the calorie deficits imposed by the diet.

The most startling result from the sirtfood diet is that muscle mass after the 1-week diet period was either the same as before, or showed slight improvements. Dieting law typically states that when losing fat, muscle is also lost, usually around 20-30% of the total weight loss, you should lose 2-3 lbs. of muscle for every 10 lbs. lost.

Of course, retaining muscle isn't just better from an overall fitness perspective, but also from an aesthetic view. A common fear, especially in men, is that if they lose weight is that they will look skinny, scrawny and unhealthy. Yet by the retaining the muscle you will gain that toned, slither look that is so fashionable in models.

Another important reason why retaining muscle mass is your resting energy expenditure. Your muscles require energy, even when you are not using them intensely. Owing to this, people who keep skeletal muscle burn more calories than people who don't, even if both people are sedentary. Basically, being muscular allows you to eat more calories and get away with it!

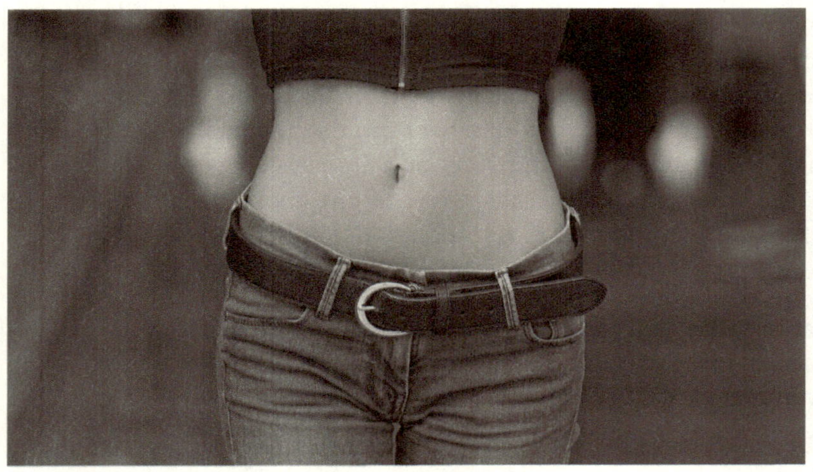

Muscle mass has also been associated with a general decrease in degenerative diseases as you age (such as diabetes and osteoporosis) as well as lower rates of mental health problems (such as depression and excessive anger).

Overall, the clinical trial performed at the fitness center not only supported the notion that the sirtfood diet can aid weight loss and promote holistic body health, but it also leads to the surprising finding that sirtfoods can retain muscle mass.

This is the beauty of the sirtfood diet it isn't trying to make your eating habits artificial and awkward. It is simply copying the healthiest practices that already exist around the world.

Skeletal muscle is all the muscles you voluntarily control, such as the muscles in your limbs, back, shoulders, and so on. There are two other types: cardiac muscle is what the heart is formed of, while the smooth muscle is your involuntary muscles which includes muscles around your blood vessels, face and various parts of organs and other tissues.

Skeletal muscle is separated into two different groups, the blandly named type-1 and type-2. Type 1 muscle is effective at continued, sustained activity whereas type-2 muscle is effective at short, intense periods of activity. So, for example, you would predominantly use type-1 muscles for jogging, but type-2 muscles for sprinting.

Sirt-1 protects the type-1 muscles, but not the type-2 muscle, which is still broken down for energy. Therefore, holistic muscle mass drops when fasting, even though type-1 skeletal muscle mass increases.

Sirt-1 also influences how the muscles work. Sirt-1 is produced by the muscle cells, but the ability to produce sirt-1 decreases as the muscle ages. As a result, muscle is harder to build as you age and doesn't grow as fast in response to exercise. A lack of sirt-1 also causes the muscles to become tired quicker and gradually decline over time.

When you start to consider these effects of sirt-1, you can start to form a picture of why fasting helps keep the body supple. Fasting releases sirt-1, which in turn helps skeletal muscle grow and stay in good shape. sirt-1 is also released by consuming sirtuin activators, giving the sirtfood diet its muscle retaining power.

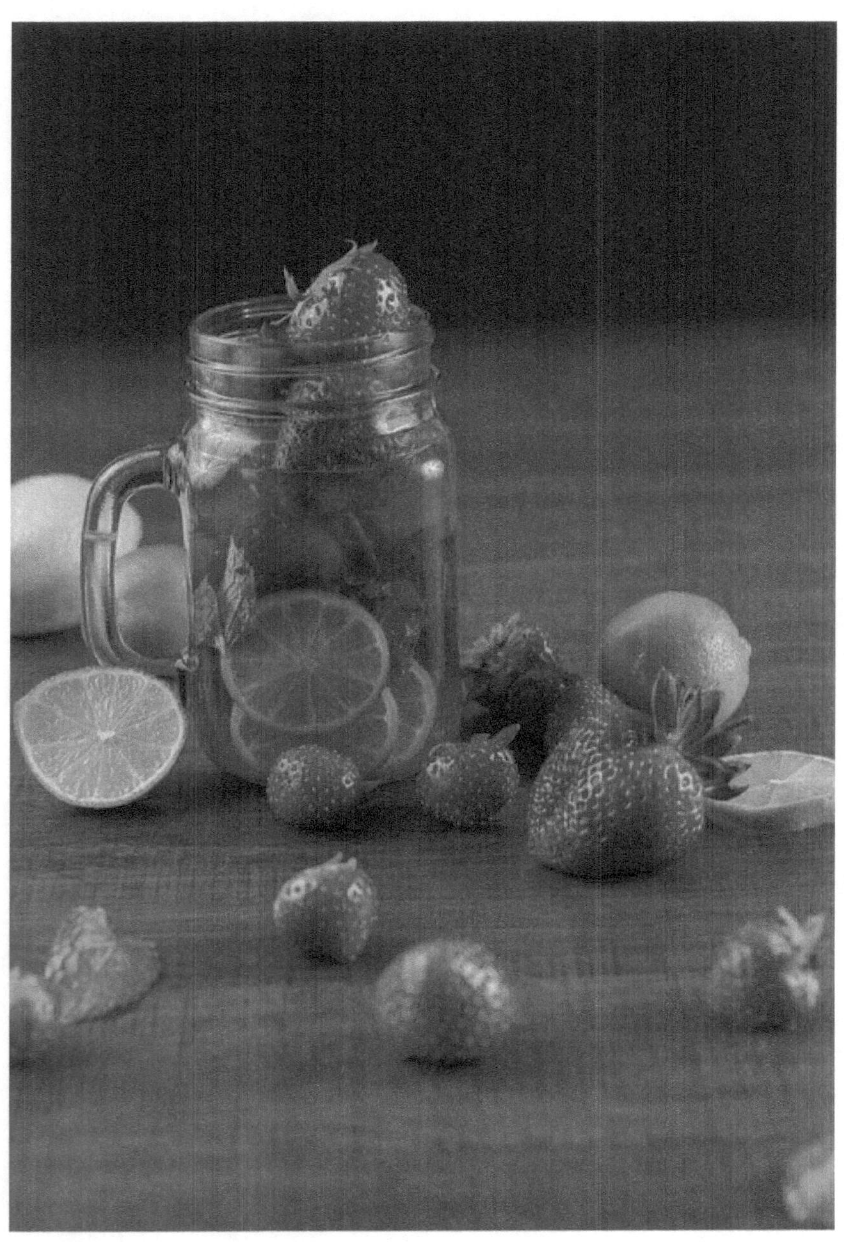

Chapter 2
How the sirtfood diet works

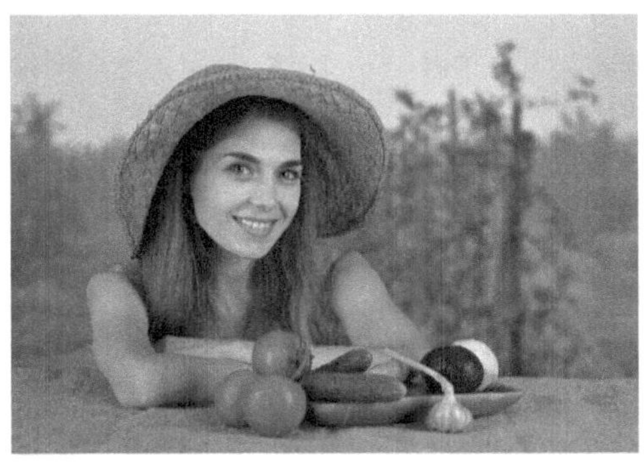

The basis of the sirtuin diet can be explained in simple terms or in complex ways. It is important to understand how and why it works however, so that you can appreciate the value of what you are doing. It is important to also know why these sirtuin rich foods help to help you maintain fidelity to your diet plan. Otherwise, you may throw something in your meal with less nutrition that would defeat the purpose of planning for one rich in sirtuins. Most importantly, this is not a dietary fad, and as you will see, there is much wisdom contained in how humans have used natural foods even for medicinal purposes, over thousands of years.

To understand how the Sirtfood diet works, and why these particular foods are necessary, we will look at the role they play in the human body.

Sirtuin activity was first researched in yeast, where a mutation caused an extension in the yeast's lifespan. Sirtuins were also shown to slow aging in laboratory mice, fruit flies, and nematodes. As research on Sirtuins proved to transfer to mammals, they were examined for their use in diet and slowing the aging process. The sirtuins in humans are different in the typing but they essentially work in the same ways and reasons.

There are seven "members" that make up the sirtuin family. It is believed that sirtuins play a big role in regulating certain functions of cells including proliferation (reproduction and growth of cells), apoptosis (death of cells). They promote survival and resist stress to increase longevity.

They are also seen to block neurodegeneration (loss or function of the nerve cells in the brain). They conduct their housekeeping functions by cleaning out toxic proteins and supporting the brain's ability to change and adapt to different conditions, or to recuperate (i.e., brain plasticity). As part of this they also help reduce chronic inflammation, and reduce something called oxidative stress. Oxidative stress is when there are too many cell-damaging free radicals circulating in the body, and the body cannot catch up by combating them with anti-oxidants. These factors are related to age-related illness and weight as well, which again, brings us back to a discussion of how they actually work.

You will see labels in Sirtuins that start with "SIR," which represents "Silence Information Regulator" genes. They do exactly that, silence or regulate, as part of their functions. The seven sirtuins that humans work with are: SIRT1, SIRT2, SIRT3, SIRT4, SIRT 5, SIRT6 and SIRT7. Each of these types is responsible for different areas of protecting cells. They work by either stimulating or turning on certain gene expressions, or by reducing and turning off other gene expressions. This essentially means that they can influence genes to do more or less of something, most of which they are already programmed to do.

Through enzyme reactions, each of the SIRT types affect different areas of cells that are responsible for the metabolic processes that help to maintain life. This is also related to what organs and functions they will affect.

For example, the SIRT6 causes an expression of genes in humans that affect skeletal muscle, fat tissue, brain, and heart. SIRT 3 would cause an expression of genes that affect the kidneys, liver, brain and heart.

If we tie these concepts together, you can see that the Sirtuin proteins can change the expression of genes, and in the case of the Sirtfood diet we care about how sirtuins can turn off those genes that are responsible for speeding up aging and for weight management.

The other aspect to this conversation of sirtuins is the function and the power of calorie restriction on the human body. Calorie restriction is simply eating less calories. This, coupled with exercise and reducing stress is usually a combination for weight loss. Calorie restriction has also proven across much research in animals and humans to increase one's lifespan.

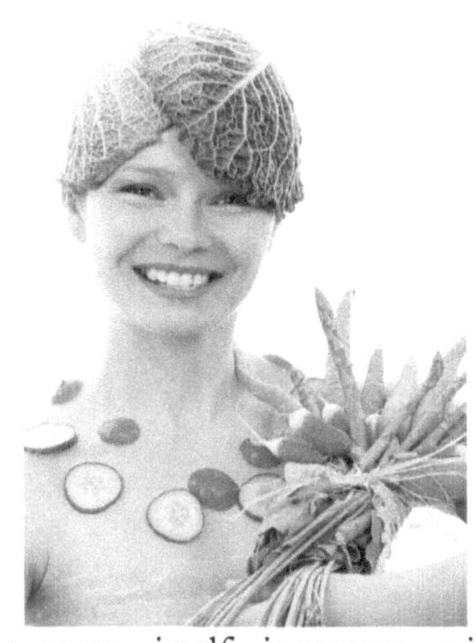

We can look further at the role of sirtuins with calorie restriction, and using the SIRT3 protein which has a role in metabolism and aging. Amongst all of the effects of the protein on gene expression, (such as preventing cells from dying, reducing tumors from growing, etc.), we want to understand the effects of SIRT3 on weight for the purpose of this book.

The SIRT3 has high expression in those metabolically active tissues as we stated earlier, and its ability to express itself increases with caloric restriction, fasting, and exercise. On the contrary, it will express itself less when the body has a high fat, high calorie-riddled diet.

The last few highlights of sirtuins are their role in regulating telomeres and reducing inflammation which also help with staving off disease and aging.

Telomeres are sequences of proteins at the ends of chromosomes. When cells divide these get shorter. As we age they get shorter, and other stressors to the body also will contribute to this. Maintaining these longer telomeres is the key to slower aging. In addition, proper diet, along with exercise and other variables can lengthen telomeres. SIRT6 is one of the sirtuins that, if activated, can help with DNA damage, inflammation and oxidative stress. SIRT1 also helps with inflammatory response cycles that are related to many age-related diseases.

Calories restriction, as we mentioned earlier, can extend life to some degree.

Since this, as well as fasting, is a stressor, these factors will stimulate the SIRT3 proteins to kick in and protect the body from the stressors and excess free radicals. Again, the telomere length is affected as well.

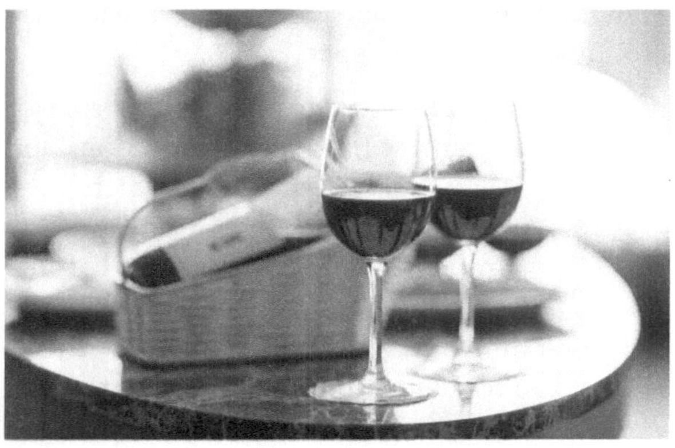

To sum up, all of this information also shows that, contrary to some people's beliefs that in terms of genetics, through our own lifestyle choices, and what we are exposed to, we can influence action and changes in our genes. This is quite an empowering thought, and yet another reason why you should be excited to have a science-based diet such as the Sirtfood diet, available to you.

Having laid this all out before you, you should be able to appreciate how and why these miraculous compounds work in your favor, to keep you youthful, healthy, and lean If they are working hard for you, don't you feel that you should do something too? Well, you can, and that is what the rest of this book will do for you.

Chapter 3: How to adhere to sirtfood diet

The Sirtfood Diet was never meant to be a quick fix or to last only for 3 weeks. It is a lifestyle.

Never Diet Again

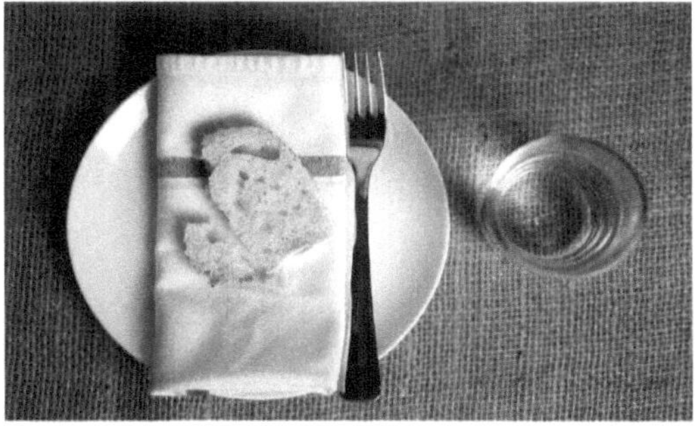

Perhaps the greatest thing about the Sirtfood Diet is the fact that if you incorporate these foods into your life on a daily basis, you will find that you never have to even think about dieting again. You will attain your goal weight with patience and dedication, and it won't come back.

Not only will you be at your ideal body weight, but you'll have more energy, clearer skin, a healthier heart, and a stronger body and you'll be happier than you can remember ever being. Such is the power of sirtuin-activating foods. From this point forward, you will not have to anguish over what you're not allowed to eat because you will be too busy choosing from the extensive list of sirtfoods and polyphenol-rich foods that your body has started to crave. You will notice that the more you eat the nutrient-dense plants that are encouraged in the Sirtfood Diet, and drink your concentrated shot of sirtuin-activating compounds in your green juice, the more your body and taste buds are going to demand you continue blessing them with such great fuel. Before you even realize it, you will see a bag of chips or a doughnut that would have made you drool in longing just a few weeks or months ago, and the thought of eating it will turn your stomach.

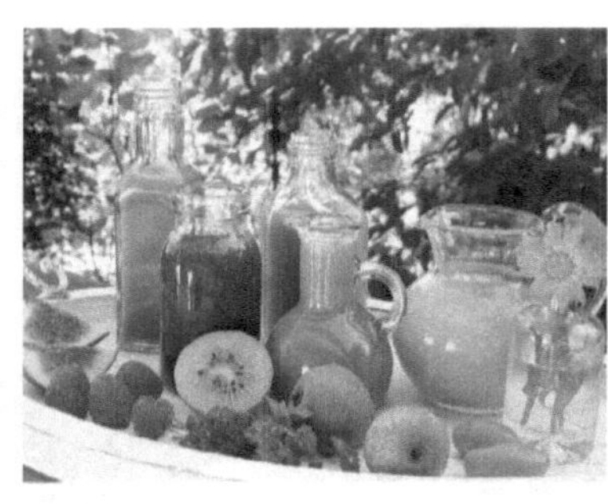

You won't be depriving yourself of the empty calories you used to binge on, you simply won't want them. There will be no room in your diet for them any longer.

There will be a learning curve as you get used to swapping out low-quality food options for nutrient-dense choices. But if you make it easy for yourself to make these choices, they will become automatic much quicker than you would believe possible.

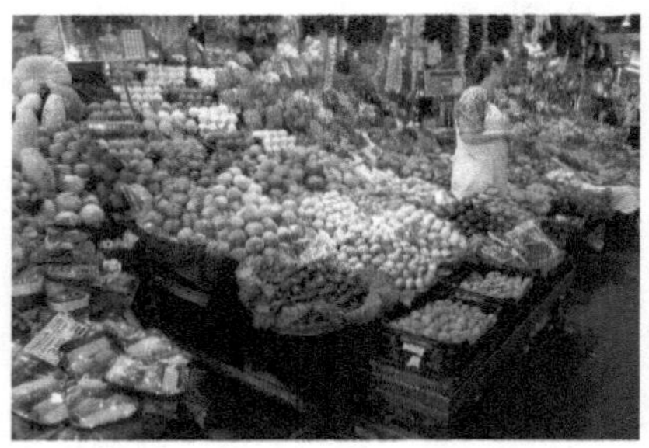

When you're shopping for your groceries, buy buckwheat pasta and whole-grain bread. Have a selection of fresh herbs, sweet and tart berries, nuts and seeds on hand to sprinkle over top of every meal. Stop buying soda and start experimenting with the different roasts of coffee, varieties of tea and, in moderation, blends of red wine.

Challenge yourself and your family members to try a new plant-based item each week, or find new ways to use the ingredients you're already comfortable with. Everything about food should be an enjoyable event, from the choosing of the highest quality ingredients to cooking with love and eating with joy. Best of all, after every meal, you won't be suffering from nagging feelings of guilt and heartburn, but instead, you'll be invigorated and proud of yourself.

There will likely be times in your life where your diet goes astray. Perhaps you go on vacation or you get injured and can't cook as much as you would like to. Maybe it's the holiday season and the power of comfort foods and nostalgic cooking overwhelmed you. Whatever the reason, acknowledge that you're human, and a setback doesn't have to hold you back or completely derail all your hard work.

Embrace a Diet of Inclusion

A very common by-product of a poor diet is a very damaged relationship with the food we eat. As a society, most of us have become very removed from the source of our food. We actively avoid learning where the animal products are coming from or how they were produced, and there are many children who are growing up unable to identify freshly harvested fruits and vegetables. They may know that carrots are orange, but they've only ever seen them cubed in pre-packed frozen or canned foods.

Because of this distance, we have lost respect for the food we're eating. For most of us, it's readily available whenever we want it, so we take it for granted. This often encourages us to overconsume, especially if we also factor in the additives that are in pre-made foods.

When we eat food that doesn't nourish us, our bodies rebel. We feel sick, tired, and unhappy. So we start to tell ourselves all the things we're not allowed to do. We can't eat our favorite cookies, and we're no longer allowed to go out for our favorite fast food. We can't have more than 800 calories a day and we can't eat any carbs/fat/sugar, etc.

All of this pressure makes us feel guilty about every morsel of food we eat, but we're so deeply engrained in the cycle that it's very difficult to tunnel our ways out without help.

Sustaining Lifestyle Changes and Choices

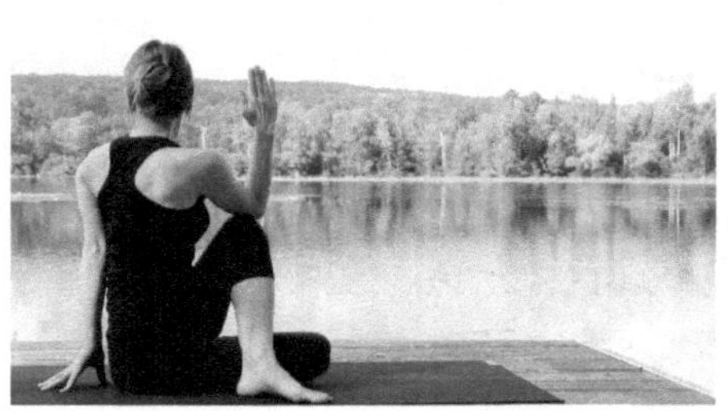

Devoting yourself to being mindful of your food choices isn't the only other change you will have to sustain in your life if you truly want to be committed to retaining your health and maintaining healthy body weight.

At the very beginning of this book, you were encouraged to let go of target weight goals and instead replace them with health goals. Good health is a lifetime achievement, with no end date. Chances are, you still kept a magic number in your mind as you kept reading this book. When you start the first 2 stages of the diet, hopefully, you'll see enough positive changes to refocus your attention on health and away from the weight aspect. If you stick to the Sirtfood Diet, however, there will come a day when you realized you've reached that magic number.

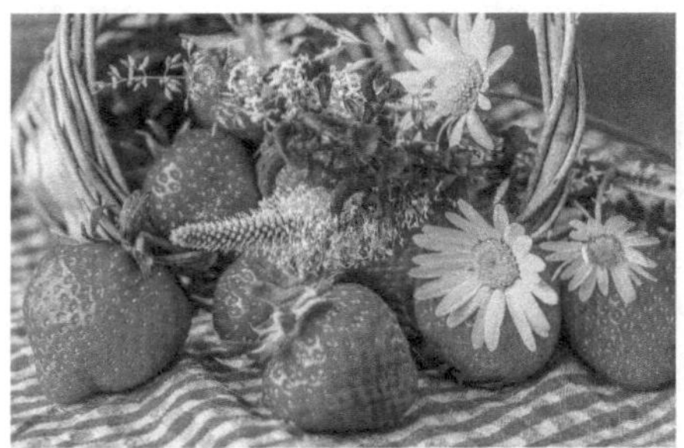

When that happens, you should celebrate your accomplishments. Having healthy body composition is an incredible indicator of health and it's something to be very proud of. But don't let this achievement affect your future success. You certainly don't have to restrict calories anymore and possibly never again, but if you want to stay healthy, you do need to continue feeding your body all the nourishment it has come to know, love and deserve. Sirtfoods are a part of your life now, and forevermore

Chapter 4: Benefits of sirtfoods

• Switching on fat burning and protection from weight gain.

Sirtuins do this by increasing the functionality of the mitochondrion (which is involved in the production of energy) and sparking a change in your metabolism to break down more fat cells. Sirts that are activated increase the amount of the neurotransmitter which is used as a signal to the fat cells. These transmitters help in telling the fat cells to breakdown and also change into energy.

• Improving memory by protecting neurons from damage.

Sirtuins also boost learning skills and memory through the enhancement of synaptic plasticity. Synaptic plasticity refers to the ability of synapses to weaken or strengthen with time due to decrease or increase in their activity. This is important because memories are represented by different interconnect network of synapses in the brain and synaptic plasticity is an important neurochemical foundation of memory and learning.

• Slowing down the ageing process.

Sirtuins act as cell guarding enzymes. Thus, they protect the cells and slow down their ageing process.

- ## Repairing cells.

  The sirtuins repair cells damaged by re-activating cell functionality.

- ## Protection against diabetes.

  This happens through prevention against insulin resistance. Sirtuins do this by controlling blood sugar levels because this diet calls for moderate consumption of carbohydrates. These foods cause increases in blood sugar levels; hence the need to release insulin and as the blood sugar levels increase greatly there is need to produce more insulin. Over time, cells become resistant to insulin; hence, the need to produce more insulin and this leads to insulin resistance.

- ## Fighting cancers.

  The chemicals working as sirtuin activators affect the function of sirtuin in different cells, i.e. By switching it on when in normal cells and shutting it down in cancerous cells. This encourages the death of cancerous cells.

- ## Fighting inflammation.

  Sirtuins have a powerful antioxidant effect that has the power to reduce oxidative stress. This has positive effects on heart health and cardiovascular protection.

- **The sirtfood diet estimates achievement just regarding weight reduction.**

Weight is a determinant of wellbeing. However, it's not alone. To gauge somebody's wellbeing accomplishment on whether they lose X pounds in X measure of time disregards the various advantages of nourishment. It additionally has supplements that can advance a few substantial capacities and is regularly a euphoric encounter established in the convention. For by and broad wellbeing, there's quite a lot more to concentrate on than fundamentally appearance, and estimating achievement just regarding weight reduction is incomprehensive.

- **It's prohibitive, which can harm your association with nourishment.**

This eating routine underlines an admission of 1,000 to 1,500 calories for every day, which is a lot of lower than the vast majority need. At the point when we severely limit our nourishment consumption, our natural response is to gorge. Your body is keen, and it thinks about this absence of sustenance as an assault. Along these lines, we will in general overcompensate, which is the reason we as a whole can identify with being "hangry" and therefore overindulging whenever we're at last allowed to eat. Rehearsing careful and natural eating is a more supportable course than confining nourishment.

- # The sirtfood diet isn't science-based.

While there is some questionable research about the advantages of sirtuins, there's practically zero research about the particular sirtfood diet. Additionally, we as of now have a few rules set up that have been altogether looked into and tried for quite a long time. In case you're lost on what "solid nourishment" is, this is a superior spot to begin.

It's beautiful if you need to consolidate a couple of sirtfoods into an eating plan. Nourishments like green tea, organic product, dim chocolate, and kale all include a spot inside a smart dieting design! In any case, holding fast to a program with such exacting pass-or-bomb prerequisites is unreasonable and could be destructive to your association with nourishment. By consolidating an eating plan that is loaded with assortment and eating carefully, you'll have the option to set up a long haul, maintainable association with nourishment.

While the Sirtfood Diet was officially announced at the beginning of 2016, "superfoods" have been making headlines since WW1 when bananas were part of a massive marketing campaign sponsored by The United Fruit Company. In more modern times, we're exposed to new so-called superfoods on a monthly, if not weekly basis.

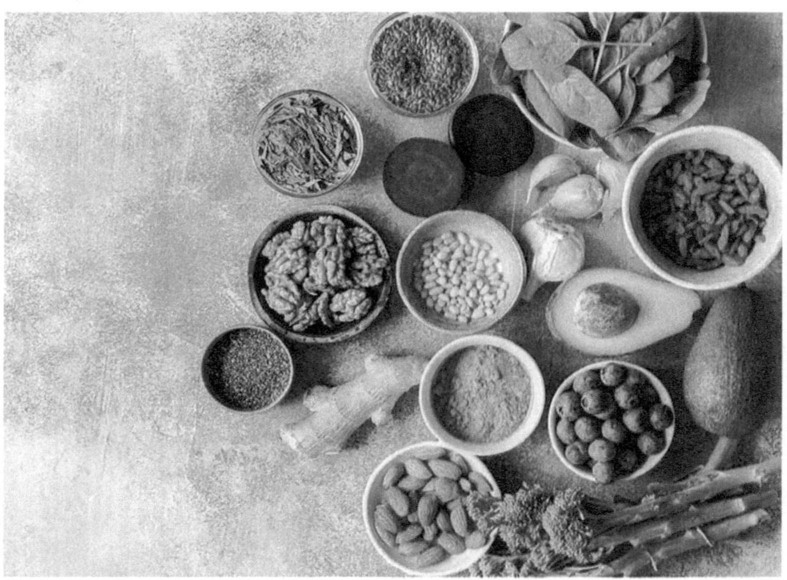

"Superfood" is not a scientific term, but rather it's a marketing gimmick. That doesn't mean there is no truth to the science behind the foods that are marketed as superfoods, or that they're not incredibly full of nutrition. It simply means that, just like a food company can use the word "natural" to mean almost anything they want it to, so can they use "superfood" as a label to promote a product.

The term Sirtfoods is not defined or regulated by a governing body either, but it logically can only be applied to foods that perform a specific scientific action: activate sirtuins.

If you're faced with a choice about whether to focus your attention on superfoods or sirtfoods, you can rest easier when you realize that most sirtfoods have, at some point, been labeled superfoods as well, so both your bases are covered.

Following a sirtfood diet, however, is designed to encourage the addition of an entire category of foods, rather than trying to overdose on the single, newest trendy superfood. A wide variety of sirtfoods should fill your plate, providing you with a constantly rotating mix of nutrients to fuel your body.

The world of medical research has been dissecting the value of plant-based food for decades, and we all know that they are good for us. They're full of vitamins, minerals, and the almighty antioxidant. Antioxidants have been the focus of much media and research attention for their apparent ability to neutralize free radicals.

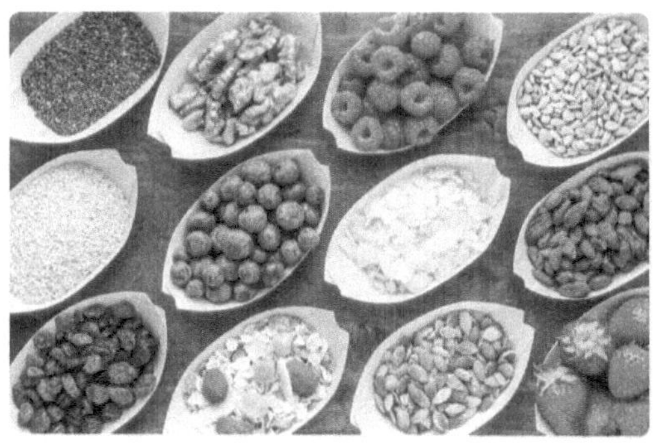

Sirtfoods, on the other hand, are life-saving for their polyphenol content, which is the sirtuin-activating compound (STAC) they got their name from. In all the latest research that follows the lifestyles and health spans of the oldest populations on earth, the common denominator is a diet rich in polyphenols. The fact that these populations are able to live high-quality lives without disease also shows that their diet must effectively protect the health of individuals of all ages.

We know that natural muscle loss begins in our 30s, if not earlier, but by activating sirtuins and living an otherwise healthy, active lifestyle, this decline can be stopped and even reversed.

There is no doubt or argument that the vitamins, minerals, and antioxidants in all edible plant-based foods are important and valuable to your health, but it is the specific polyphenols in sirtfoods that can protect, fortify and rebuild your cells on an individual level. We know it is the exceptionally high polyphenol count in foods like dark chocolate, green tea, and turmeric that fight inflammation and lower the risk of almost all chronic diseases.

Superfoods are easy to popularize and can be picked and chosen for their marketability, regardless of their true value and impact to your health. Sirtfoods are valued specifically because of their proven, scientific value to your health. Many of them overlap and they are all delicious in their own unique ways. You will find a list of the Top 20 Sirtfoods in Appendix 1 at the back of the book, as well as a list of the Top 100 Foods Rich in Polyphenols, in Appendix 2.

The majority of these foods, especially those on the top 20 list, are common ingredients that you can easily find in most supermarkets or, at the very least, online.

They're not necessarily expensive and they don't have to take over your entire meal. In many cases, they simply enhance what you already enjoy cooking and eating. Instead of focusing your attention on a new, trendy superfood each week, start a habit of including a wide variety of sirtfoods in your diet.

An habit like that can and should last the rest of your life.

Chapter 6:
The science of sirtuins – fight fat, build muscle mass, anti-aging effect

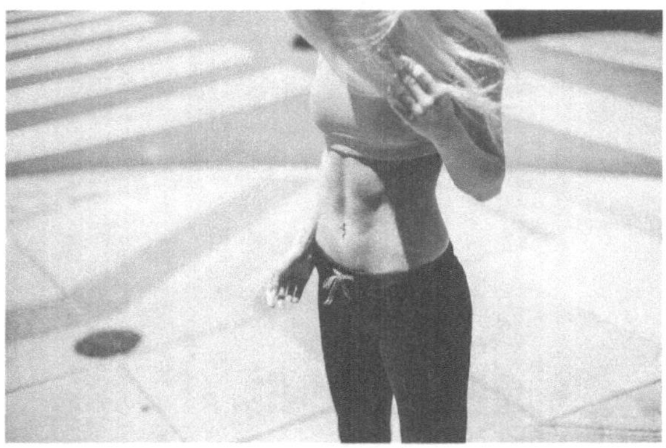

There are multiple types and classes of sirtuins that are referred to on the Sirt diet. The first class is generally simply referred to as "sirtuins," which are those found within the human body. However, when sirtuins are found in plants, which are then consumed and can be used by people, they are known as "polyphenols." These polyphenols are organic and bioactive compounds that, while a little different from the sirtuins naturally found within humans, still result in the same biochemical process that results in increased weight loss and promote a variety of health improvements.

We will now explore how sirtuins and polyphenols affect the human body and what science has proven about its benefits.

Cellular homeostasis is incredibly important for every aspect of human health. When your cells are in a state of homeostasis, it means that they are working as they should be.

They are comfortable, healthy, and doing their job appropriately. They are neither underworking or overworking; everything is as it should be.

When you are in cellular homeostasis, you naturally reduce excessive aging or illnesses, instead of promoting whole-body healing and wellness. A 2016 research study by Polish experts on biology, biochemistry, and plant physiology found that sirtuins play a key role in the process of cellular homeostasis, and it shouldn't be underestimated.

Let's go over some of the details of this pioneering study.

Don't worry; I will skip the scientific gibberish and speak in layman's terms. Both humans and plants have cellular enzymes that act as a sensor to detect and promote homeostasis.

There are different classes of these enzymes, and the third type has been dubbed "sirtuins." Not only are there two different classes of sirtuins, as we previously mentioned, there are also seven different types. These types are known simply as Sirt[number 1-7]. Each of these types has one of three roles so that they can all work together throughout the entire body.

One of the roles of some of the sirtuins is to affect the mitochondrial system. This is important, as the mitochondrial system affects a person's weight loss, healing ability, energy levels, and more. Mitochondria are known as a powerhouse.

The mitochondrial systems are one of the most important aspects of maintaining homeostasis, as, without it, no human would be able to survive. Those who live with mitochondrial dysfunctions experience severe and widespread symptoms that interfere with daily life. Thankfully, this study found that sirtuins can promote a healthy mitochondrial system leading to cellular homeostasis.

In particular, this can help a person increase metabolism and weight loss, reduce inflammation levels, lessen oxidative stress and cellular damage that lead to disease, and promote cellular longevity as you age. As you can imagine, by using sirtuins to activate the mitochondrial system, you not only can help manage and possibly treat mitochondrial disorders, but also other conditions such as obesity, type II diabetes, neurodegenerative diseases, cancer, and more.

In part, this positive change is due to the way sirtuins are able to stimulate the mitochondria and mitochondrial proteins to prevent negative changes before they can even occur and treat them directly at the source.

Polyphenols come in a number of classifications with resveratrol and quercetin, being two of them that are more widely known. Each type can have different positive effects, meaning you want to consume sirtuins from a variety of plant-based foods to experience all of the benefits. For instance, you might have heard about resveratrol being found in grape skins and therefore wine, this resveratrol is the very same sirtuins you will be consuming on the Sirt diet. This type of sirtuin specifically has been found to positively affect the Sirt1 category within the body, leading to weight loss, reduced insulin resistance, and improved motor function.

When studying polyphenols, the researchers tracked the number of polyphenols in a given serving for plant matter and their class. For instance, the classes of polyphenols tested include flavonols, flavones, isoflavones, and more. While the researchers in this specific study were unable to test all of the high-sirtuin foods that we mentioned in chapter one, the ones they did test reinforced what had already been proven: these foods are some of the highest in sirtuin and therefore perfect for the Sirt diet. Some other foods that the researchers proved her high in sirtuins and therefore helpful to consume more of include orange, lemon, grapefruit, eggplant, beans, blackberries, black currants, black grapes, cherries, and rhubarb.

It was also found that other foods and polyphenols can affect each other and how effectively your body absorbs and utilizes them. For instance, if you consume protein (such as meat) and polyphenols together, your body will be unable to absorb either the protein or the polyphenols, as well as it usually would. For this reason, it is a good idea to drink your green juice separately from your meals. It is still beneficial to add as many Sirtfoods to your meals as possible, even when you are eating protein, but just know that your body will not absorb as many of the sirtuins as it otherwise would. But, if you drink your green juice a couple of hours prior or after you consume protein, you will be able to ensure you get the most benefit out of it possible.

Similarly, the study also found that by heating plants through boiling, steaming, roasting, or cooking in any other way, the sirtuins and their benefits are reduced. Again, this doesn't mean you can't ever cook sirtuin-rich food, but should stay mindful of this and try to eat as many of them raw as possible.

The study concluded that sirtuins are incredibly powerful for general health and wellness, but people should keep in mind how what you consume them with and how you prepare them will affect the sirtuin levels within the food.

When you reduce caloric intake, it results in your metabolic and autophagy processes increasing. However, calorie reduction is not the only way you can experience this benefit, as a study published in Cell Death and Disease in 2010 found. This study found that when you activate your body's natural sirtuins through ingesting polyphenols, you can make use of these same important biological processes, which the researchers could be used to treat cancer in the future. Now, imagine, what if you combine caloric restriction along with increased polyphenol intake? It is likely that by combining these two aspects, both key aspects of the Sirt diet, you could compound the effects for even better results.

By restricting your calories and increasing your Sirt food intake, you can slow down the rate of cellular aging, thereby increasing not only the lifespan of your cells but possibly increase your own life span, as well. Not only that, but as it promotes overall health and wellness, and not simply living to an older age, you might be able to enjoy your golden years happier and healthier, living them to the fullest. Of course, no scientist or doctor, will guarantee you this, and neither will I, as anyone who makes such claims is only making false promises. Yet, I can promise you that science is on the side of Sirtuins and balanced calorie restriction. Study after study has found that both of these elements of the Sirt diet can increase a person's overall health and expected lifespan.

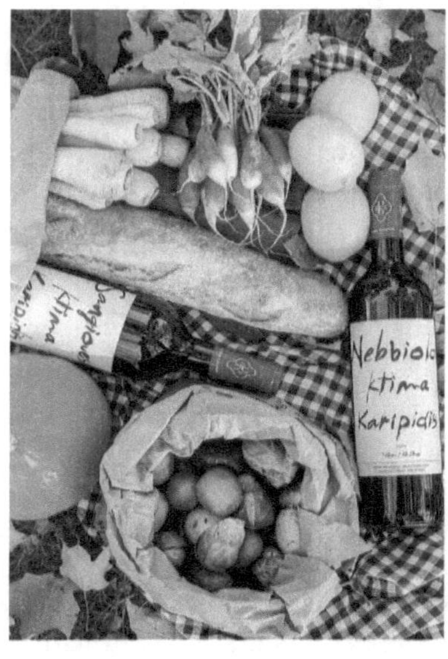

Many people have never heard of the autophagy process, despite its importance. It is a natural biochemical process of the body. Throughout human history, people have unknowingly made use of the autophagy process to help treat disease. They did this largely through fasting. Thankfully, in recent years researchers have learned more about autophagy, not only about its importance but also how we can better make use of it. No longer do we have to fast whenever we want to use this natural reaction, we can use other methods, such as calorie restriction paired with Sirt food intake, to induce it, as well.

The word "autophagy is derived from Latin, with two words combining to literally translate to "self-eating." At first appearance, it may sound like a bad idea to have your body eat itself, but I promise you, in this case, it is something you want to happen. It doesn't hurt you or damages your health. Quite the contrary, if you want to stay healthy, then your body must make use of the autophagy process.

This revolutionary process allows the body to take its damaged and dying cells and recycle them into healthier and younger cells. To put it simply, the autophagy process works similarly to compost. When you are gardening, you get rid of your old useless scraps and molded or rotting produce you are unable to use. But, instead of simply throwing these scraps into the trash, you recycle them into compost to grow new and healthier produce. It is a life cycle that continuously feeds itself so that your garden begins to flourish more day by day, and nothing goes to waste. Your body uses autophagy for the same purpose.

By utilizing the autophagy process, you can help your body to maintain a state of homeostasis, where your cells are consistently being cleaned and repaired. This is especially important in today's day in age when many of us are being assaulted by toxins from every angle. These toxins are in the food we eat, the air we breathe, and the water we drink. Not only are they coming from the outside in, but our own bodies will also produce these toxins when we don't sleep well or make other poor lifestyle choices. Autophagy helps to remove these toxins and reset your body to what it should be.

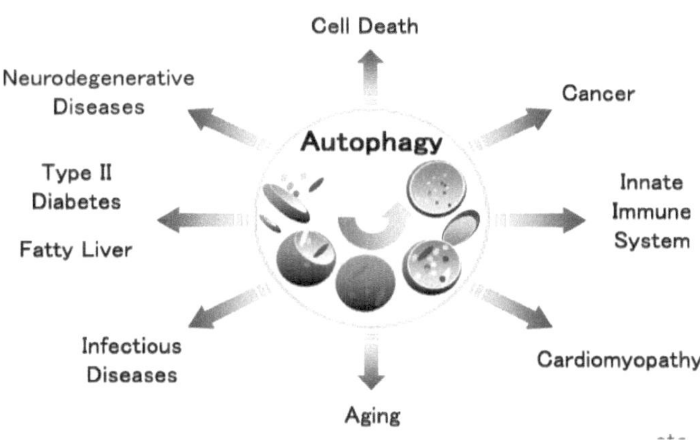

The main benefits of autophagy include reducing aging and increasing longevity. As the process literally replaces old cells with younger cells, it naturally lessens the rate of aging throughout your entire body and mind. Other benefits include recycling proteins, sorting out and removing toxins that cause neurodegenerative diseases such as Alzheimer's, and increased energy. With all of these benefits, autophagy is currently receiving a lot of attention in the scientific community, as it has a lot of potential in treating some of our most troubling diseases, such as cancer.

Many researchers are attempting to find a way to utilize autophagy in the form of a pill to target especially difficult diseases. While this research might still have a long way to go before it is on the market for cancer treatment, in the meantime, you can make use of autophagy in preventing and managing a number of diseases by promoting the process through the Sirt diet. These beneficial effects were well-documented in the 2010 study we previously mentioned.

A study published in 2017 examined why cinnamon is so powerful in improving the insulin response and blood glucose levels, both of which are important for anyone who has diabetes. It is also important for those at a heavier weight, making them predisposed to insulin resistance and high blood sugar. While scientists have long known that cinnamon has a positive effect on this aspect of health, as it has been used for healing ever since ancient times, it has long been a mystery as to why. However, with a new understanding of sirtuins, researchers decided to see if the polyphenol contents within cinnamon were to thank for these powerful healing properties.

The study found that sure enough, cinnamon is full of a number of different types of polyphenols, which are now believed to be the source of positive effects on insulin and blood sugar.

- What does this mean?

Not only can cinnamon help you, but it means that simply by increasing your overall Sirtfood intake, whether with cinnamon or any of the others listed in chapter one, you can improve your health. In order to validate this hypothesis, scientists tested the polyphenol that is found within cinnamon against the polyphenol resveratrol, which is found within grape skin and red wine.

Sure enough, scientists found that both types of polyphenols are able to positively affect insulin and blood sugar levels.

This confirmed their suspicion that the positive effects of cinnamon are a direct result of consuming polyphenols. However, it is important that I mention that the type of polyphenols found within cinnamon was generally more effective in managing blood sugar and insulin than the polyphenols found within red wine.

This is always important to remember, as you cannot rely on polyphenols from a single food source to experience the benefits from the Sirt diet, you must eat a balanced Sirt diet with as many sirtuin-rich foods as possible.

The Journal of Nutrition (in 2007) published a study focused specifically on cancer prevention by utilizing plant-based polyphenols. This study focused on the flavonoid class of polyphenol sirtuins. Within the flavonoid class are several subclasses, including:

- Flavones found withing peppers and herbs

- Isoflavones in soy

- Flavanones found in citrus fruits

- Flavanols in tea leaves

- Flavonols found in onions

- Anthocyanidins residing within grapes and berries

All of these subclasses of flavonoids have long been shown to improve overall cardio health and reduce the risk of heart disease, heart attack, stroke, high blood pressure, high cholesterol, and more. Because of these well-known benefits, the researchers of this study were interested in other ways in which flavonoids and polyphenols, in general, may help protect against disease, such as neurodegenerative diseases, rapid aging, and yes, cancer.

In order to examine how these polyphenols work together to fight cancer, the researchers examined how different forms of sirtuin-rich teas affected tumor cells. The results found that certain polyphenols have a synergistic effect when working together, making the effects more powerful than either alone. For instance, green tea and white tea are more effective when combined than when alone. More research is needed to understand all of the different synergistic effects of the various types of polyphenols, but the known results are encouraging. We may not yet know which specific polyphenols synergistically work in cohesion, but we do know that they are more powerful when combined than when alone.

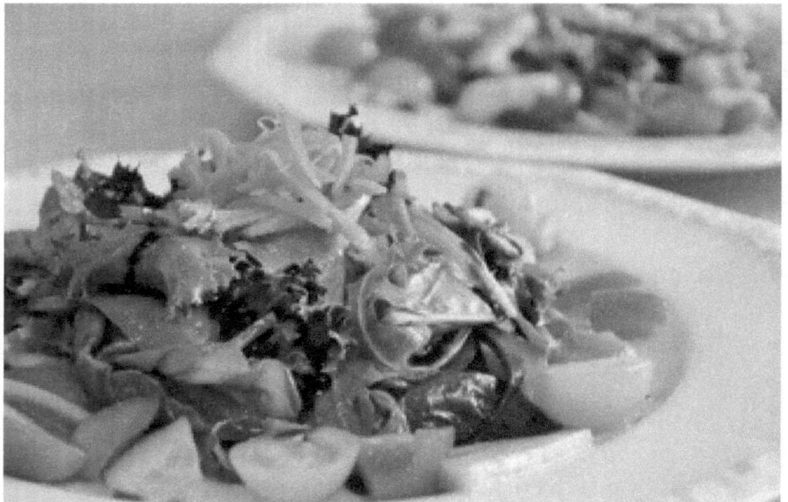

This goes to show why the Sirt green juice is so powerful: instead of getting polyphenols from a single source of plant matter, you are combining many different sources of Sirtfoods to get a wide array of polyphenol classes and subclasses.

Chapter 7: What is the skinny gene

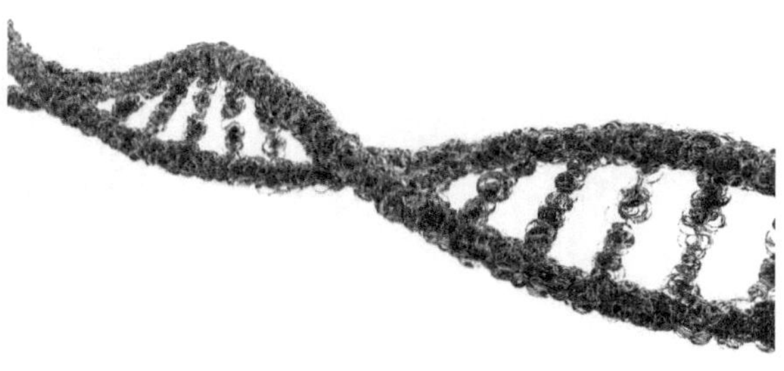

The skinny gene-diet is not difficult to follow and is divided into two phases.

The first phase lasts 7 days and is more restrictive and difficult, especially for the first 3 days. To be able to lose 3 kg every week as this diet promises, it is recommended, initially, not to exceed 1,000 calories per day in the first three days, drinking three green juices based on sirtuin-rich foods and eating only one solid meal of your choice, prepared using the ingredients indicated above.

From Day 4 to Day 7, instead, you can ingest 1,500 calories each day by taking two solid meals composed of foods rich in sirtuins and three green juices.

The sirtfood diet also called the skinny gene-diet, is the result of the studies of the two nutritionists Aidan Goggins and Glenn Matten. Their food prog, published in a volume that explains its principles and functioning, has attracted the attention of VIPs and athletes. Its effectiveness is based on the consumption of foods that stimulate sirtuins. As the creators of the diet of the moment explain, it is a family of genes present in each of us. They affect the ability to burn fat in addition to mood and the mechanisms that regulate longevity. It is no coincidence that they are also called "super metabolic regulators." Recent studies have shown that several foods can stimulate sirtuins. Their consumption would, therefore, allow them to activate the metabolism and lose weight without having to undergo extreme diets.

What makes the sirtfood diet different from the others is its "inclusion" philosophy. In fact, it is not based on the total or partial exclusion of some foods from your diet. Rather, it suggests which foods should be added to lose weight more easily. In this way, you will no longer have to undergo excessive deprivation or exhausting willpower. And you won't have to resort to expensive supplements or products with mysterious components. By eating a balanced diet and supporting it, if desired, with proper physical activity, according to the two nutritionists, you can lose about 3.5kg in a week.

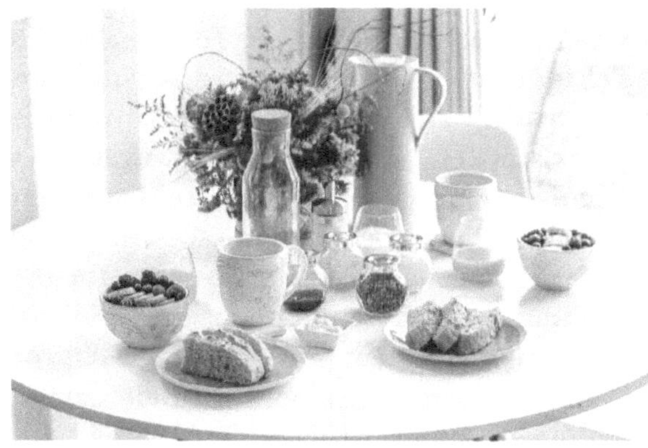

Sirtfoods became famous thanks to an important study conducted in 2003, during which scientists analyzed a particular substance, resveratrol, present in the peel of black grapes, red wine, and yeast, which would produce the same effects of calorie restriction without need to decrease your daily calories intake. Later, researchers found that other substances in red wine had a similar effect, which would explain the benefits of consuming this drink and why those who consume it get less fat.

This naturally stimulated the search for other foods containing a high concentration of these nutrients, capable of producing such a beneficial effect on the body, and studies gradually discovered several. If some are almost unknown, such as lovage, an herb that is by now very little used in cooking, the great majority is represented by well-known and widely used foods.

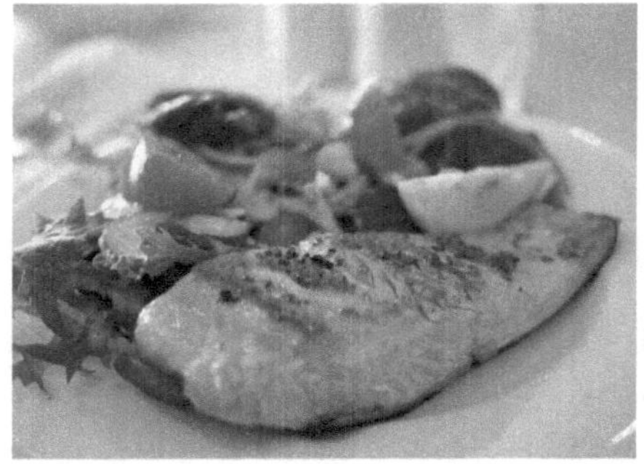

After the discovery in 2003, the enthusiasm for the benefits of sort's food skyrocketed. Studies revealed that these foods don't just mimic the calorie restriction effects. They also act as super regulators of the entire metabolism: they burn fat, increase muscle mass, and improve the health of our cells.

The world of medical research was close to the most important nutritional discovery of the century. Unfortunately, a mistake was made: the pharmaceutical industry invested hundreds of millions of pounds in an attempt to turn sirt foods into a sort of miracle pill, and the diet took a back seat. The sirtfood diet, however, does not share this pharmaceutical approach, which seeks (so far without result) to concentrate the gains from these compound nutrients of plant origin into one drug. Instead of waiting for the pharmaceutical industry to transform the nutrients of the foods we eat into a miraculous product (which may not work anyway), the sirtfood diet consists of eating these substances in their natural form that of food, to take full advantage of them. This is the basis of the pilot experiment of the sirtfood diet, with which the creators intended to create a diet containing the richest sources of sirt foods and observe their effects.

During their studies, Glen Matten and Aidan Goggins discovered that the best sirt foods are consumed regularly by populations who boast the least incidence of diseases and obesity on earth.

The Kuna Indians, in the American continent, seem immune from hypertension and with very low levels of cancer, diabetes, obesity, and early death thanks to the intake of cocoa, excellent sirt food. In Okinawa, Japan, sirt food, dry physique, and longevity go hand in hand.

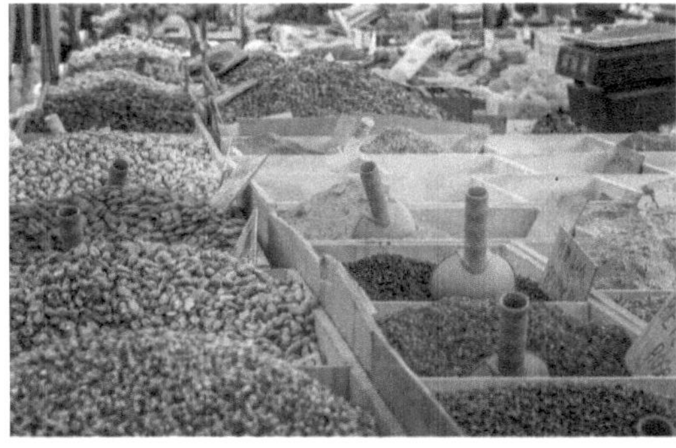

In India, the passion for spicy foods, especially turmeric, gives good results in the fight against cancer. And in the traditional Mediterranean diet, which the rest of the western world envies, chronic diseases are the exception, and obesity is contained, not the custom. Wild green leafy vegetables, dates, aromatic herbs, berries, extra virgin olive oil, red wine, and dried fruits are all effective sirt foods, and they are all present in the Mediterranean diet.

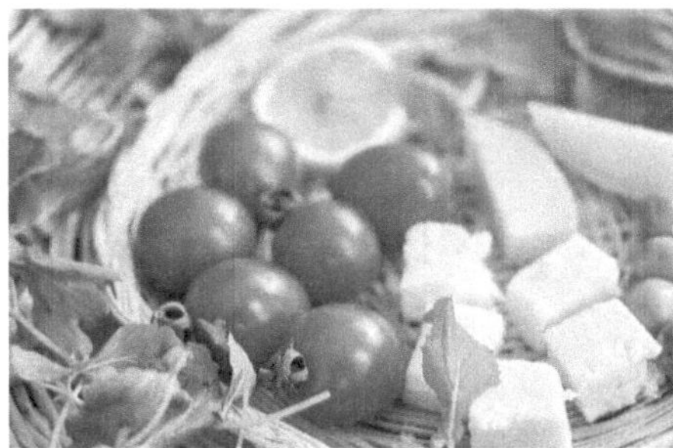

The scientific world has had to surrender to the evidence: it seems that the Mediterranean diet is more effective than reducing calories to lose weight and more effective than drugs to eliminate diseases.

Although sirt foods are not a backbone of nutrition in most of the western world today, the situation was quite different in the past. They were a basic element, and if many have become rare and others have even disappeared, it is definitely possible to reverse the course of this.

The good news is that you don't have to be a top athlete, and not even sporty, to enjoy the same benefits. We took advantage of everything we learned about sirt foods thanks to the pilot study by and the work done with sportsmen, and we adapted it to create a diet suitable for anyone who wants to lose weight while improving health.

It is not necessary to practice unsustainable fasting or to undergo endless sessions in the gym (although, of course, practicing a little physical activity would be good for you). It is not an expensive diet, nor will it waste your time, and all the foods recommended in the diet are readily available. The only accessory you will need is an extractor or centrifuge. Unlike other diets, which tell you what to eliminate, this diet tells you what to eat.

Generally, you can eat foods that are high in protein and low in fat. Among the meat-based recipes, you can choose, for example, chicken with red onion and black cabbage, turkey with cauliflower couscous, turkey escalope with capers and parsley. For fish dishes, sautéed salmon fillet, sautéed prawns, or baked marinated cod are fine.

Recipes of side dishes, light and tasty, can be prepared with beans, lentils, aubergines cut into wedges, and cooked in the oven, Walldorf salad, or red onions. And as for dessert, you can eat delicious and healthy strawberries, with a very high content of sirtuins. Plus, remember that 15-20g of dark chocolate are allowed every day.

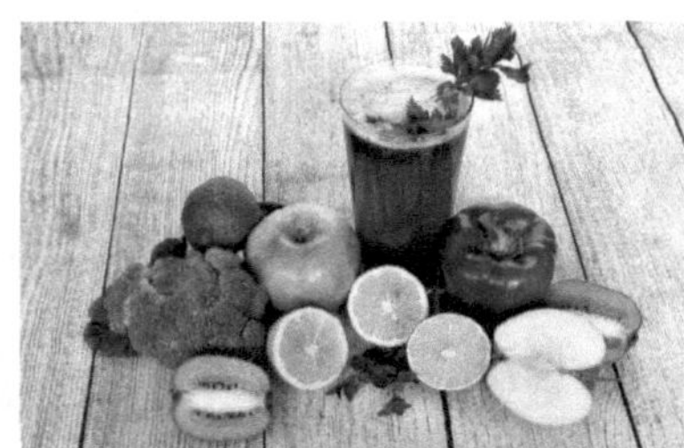

The green juice is an important part of the diet, because it has the ability to cleanse and detoxify, and will be the protagonist in the first week of the sirt prog.
Sirt foods are particularly rich in special nutrients of plant origin recently discovered, which, stimulated by fasting, activate the genes of thinness.

The foods suggested in the sirtfood diet are fresh, genuine and easily available, such as extra virgin olive oil, dark chocolate, citrus fruits, strawberries, apples, cabbage, celery, spinach, buckwheat, blueberries, nuts, soya beans, rocket salad, red onion, coffee, green tea, red wine, chili pepper, tofu, turmeric, and dates.

In addition, combined with each other or with other foods, they allow you to create very tasty dishes.

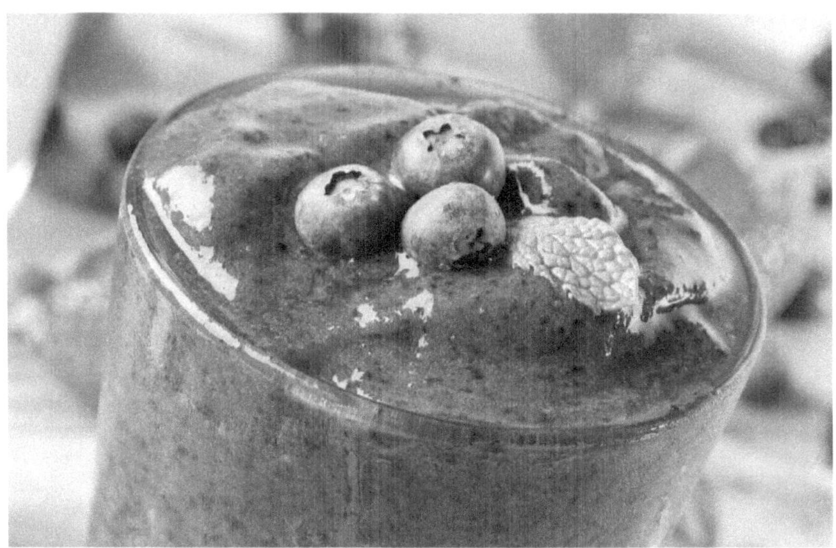

Chapter 8:
How to follow the sirtfood diet

During the first three days, the intake of calories will have to be limited to 1,000 per day at most. You can have three green juices and a solid meal, all based on sirt foods. From day 4 to 7, the daily calories will become fifteen hundred. Every day you will eat two green juices and two solid sirt meals. By the end of the seven days, you should have lost, on average, 3.5kg.

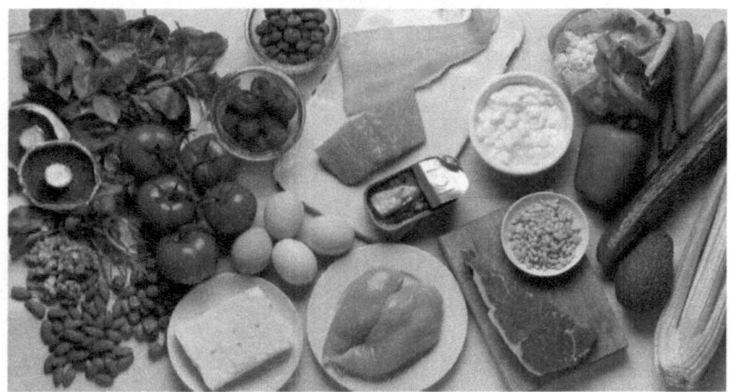

Despite the reduction in calories, the participants do not feel hungry, and the calorie limit is an indication rather than a goal. Even in the most intensive phase, calorie restriction is not as drastic as in many other regimes. Sirt foods have a naturally satiating effect so that many of you will feel pleasantly full and satisfied.

Phase 2 is the maintenance phase and lasts 14 days: during this period, although the main objective is not the reduction of calories, you will consolidate weight loss and continue to lose weight. The secret to succeeding at this stage lies in continuing to eat sirt foods in abundance; following the prog that we will provide you with relative recipes will facilitate you. During those two weeks, you will consume three balanced and rich sirt foods per day and a green sirt juice.

The procedure of the sirtfood diet

The sirt food diet consists of three phases: in phase one, the body is relieved as with a gentle fast. In the second phase, you lose pounds; in the third phase, you keep the desired weight.

Sometimes two phases are spoken of, in which case the first phase consists of phase 1 and 2.

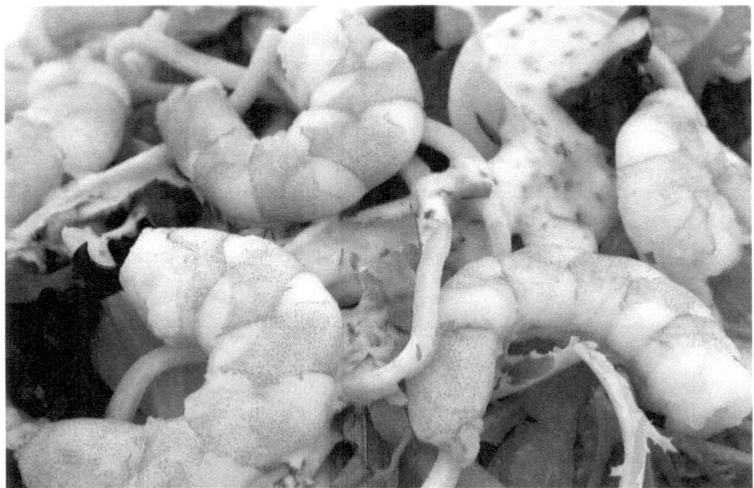

You can repeat these three phases as often as you want to lose weight. However, we recommend that you continue to "sirtify" your diet after these phases are complete by regularly including sirt foods in your meals. We also recommend that you continue drinking green juice or smoothies every day.

The 3 phases of the sirtfood diet:

- **Phase 1**

The first phase is the reprogramming of the metabolism to "lean". This works, for example, with sirtuin-rich green juices that detoxify the body. It lasts for three days. This means 1,000 calories per day in the form of 3 juices and 1 main meal.

- **Phase 2**

The calorie intake is increased to 1,500 calories. It lasts for four days. There are now 2 green juices and 2 main meals per day.

- **Phase 3**

serves to stabilise the new weight. In the third or "maintenance" phase, everything is allowed as long as you have as many sirt foods on the menu as possible and eat about 1800 calories. It lasts for two weeks. There are 1 green juice and 3 main meals per day.

You should drink the juice first, about 30 minutes before breakfast. The dinner should be taken until 7 pm if possible. You should drink water, green tea or black coffee. Black or white tea is also fine. Red wine is also allowed, but not more than two to three glasses per week, otherwise the fat will be stored again.

Chapter 9: The top sirtfood

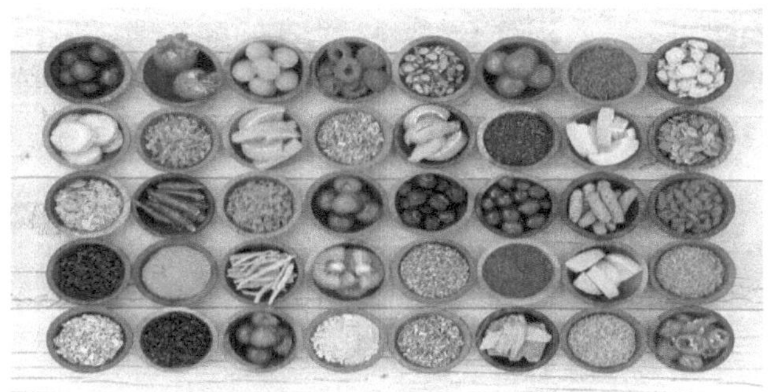

- **Arugula**

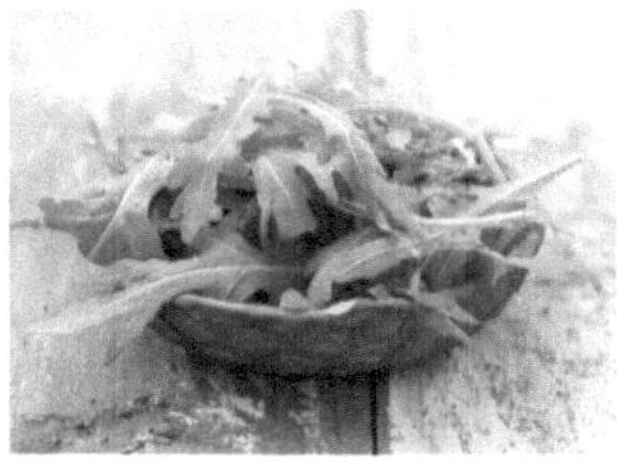

This green salad leaf (also known as rucola) is very common in the Mediterranean diet. It is not too popular in the US food culture, and it is considered an absolute arrogance to have it on your plate. However, we're not talking about a leaf covered in gold or silver; we're talking about a green salad leaf with a peppery taste that can be used for digestive and diuretic purposes. During the time of ancient Rome and in the Middle Ages, this leaf was known to have aphrodisiac properties. However, there's a lot more to this miracle leaf. It has nutrients like quercetin and kaempferol capable of activating sirtuins. This combination is said to have very positive effects on the skin as it can moisturize and improve collagen synthesis. So why not have this leaf in your salad and add some extra olive oil on it, making it a powerful sirtfood duo? As you can see, it has a lot of positive effects on your body.

- Buckwheat

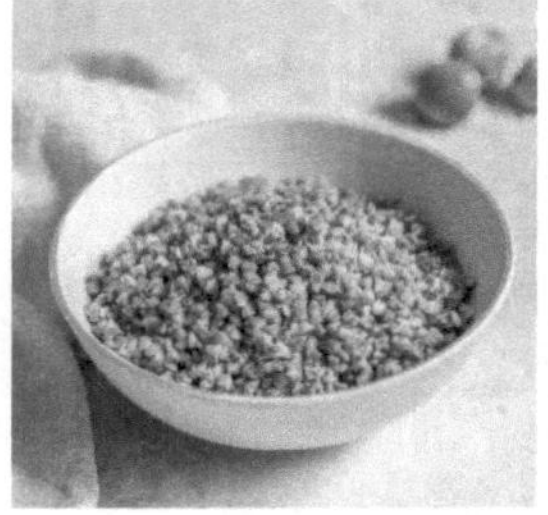

This is one of the best sources for rutin, a sirtuin-activator nutrient. However, this crop is also amazing for ecological and sustainable farming, as it can improve the quality of the soil and prevent weed growth. However, probably the most interesting part about buckwheat is that it is a fruit seed, kind of like rhubarb, so it is not a grain at all. There isn't a coincidence at all that buckwheat has more protein than any grain known to man, so it fits perfectly in your sirtfood diet. For every person trying to avoid gluten, this can be the ideal food. It is the ideal alternative for grains.

- Capers

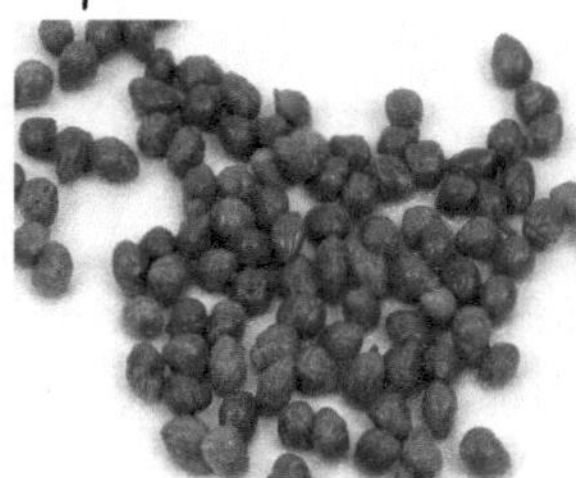

Some of you may not be too familiar with capers. If you haven't had the chance to taste them, you should. They are those dark-green salty things you can see sometimes on top of a pizza. Unfortunately, capers are not very used in a standard diet (it is very overlooked and underrated), but those who never had the chance to try capers don't know what they are missing. We are talking about the flower buds of the caper bush, a plant growing abundantly in the Mediterranean region. It is usually handpicked and preserved, and it has some interesting antidiabetic, anti-inflammatory, antimicrobial, antiviral, and immunomodulatory properties. Moreover, it has been used in medicine all around the Mediterranean area.

Capers are also rich in sirtuin-activating nutrients, so they have the chance to shine in the sirtfood diet, and I can guarantee that you will fall in love with them.

- Celery

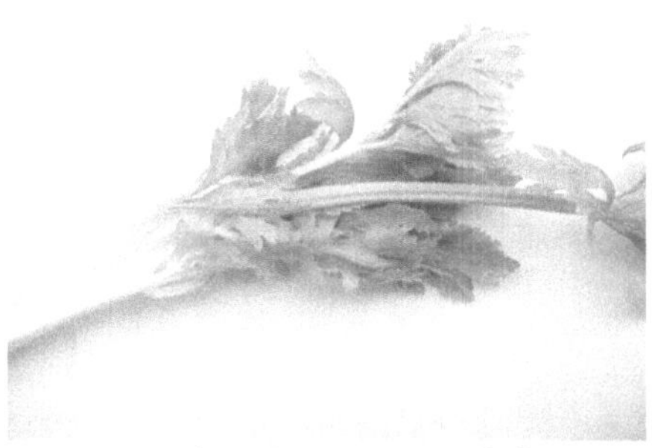

This is a plant used for thousands of years, as in ancient Egypt people were already aware of it and its properties. Back then, it was considered a medicinal plant that can be used for detoxing, cleansing, and preventing diseases. Therefore, celery consumption is very good for your gut, kidney, and liver. When it was growing wildly in ancient times, it had a strong bitter flavor. However, ever since its domestication in the 17th century, celery has become a bit sweeter, and now it can be used in salads.

There are two types of celery:

- Pascal (green)
- Blanched (yellow).

Blanching is the technique used to reduce celery's bitter taste (too strong by many standards) by shading the plant from sunlight before harvesting. This leads to a milder flavor and a paler color. Unfortunately, the blanched celery is not the version you want if you want to reap the full benefits of this plant.

Luckily, the trend is changing, and more and more people are willing to try the green celery even though its taste is very bitter. This is the type I would recommend, as it contains plenty of nutrients to activate sirtuins. It may have a bitter taste, but you can use it in salads and green juices as well.

Keep in mind that the most nutritious parts are the leaves and the hearts.

- ## Chilies

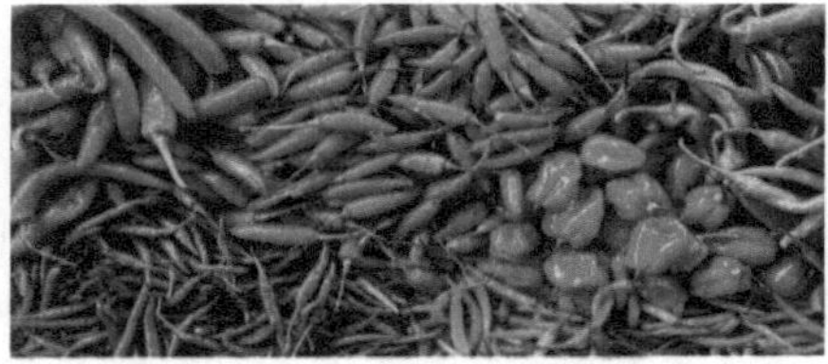

This veggie should be in your diet whether you like eating spicy food or not. It contains capsaicin, and this substance makes us savor it even more. Consuming chilies is great for activating sirtuins and it speeds up your metabolism. In fact, the spicier the chili is, the more powerful it is when it comes to activating sirtuins. You probably heard that people eating spicy food three or four times per week have a 14 percent lower death rate compared to people who eat them less than once a week. Now, this doesn't mean that you have to go for the hottest chilies you can find, especially if you are not a spicy food enthusiast. Take it easy at the beginning. You can consume Serrano peppers and then work yourself to spicier pepper. Thai chilies are very spicy, so they have a maximum sirtuin-activating effect. But to get there, you have to take it easy. Slowly work yourself to the top. When buying these peppers, make sure you select the fresh ones with deep colors. You need to avoid the soft and wrinkled ones.

- ## Cocoa

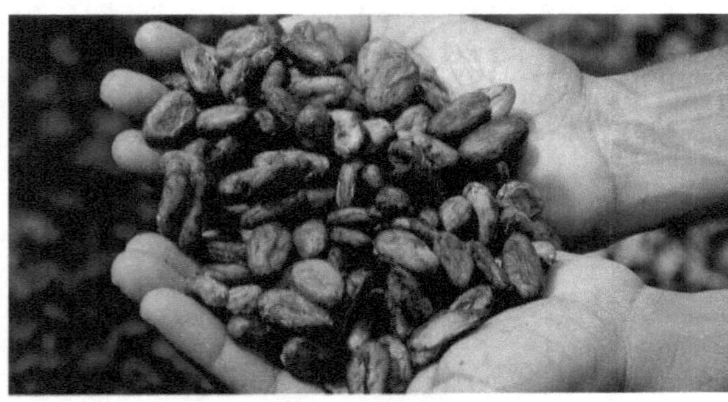

Cocoa was considered sacred by the Aztecs and Mayans, and it was a food type reserved only for the warriors or the elite. It was often used as a currency, as people were aware of its value. Although back then it was mostly used as a drink, you don't have to dilute it with milk or water to reap the full benefits of it. The best way to consume cocoa is by eating dark chocolate (with at least 85 percent solid cocoa). However, this also depends on how the chocolate is made, as this product is usually treated with an alkalizing agent, which is known to lower the acidity of the chocolate and give a darker color. This substance is also known to reduce the sirtuin-activating flavanols. In the United States, food treated with this agent is properly labeled, but this measure doesn't apply worldwide. Most countries don't have such legislation to force food processors to label their products "processed with alkali." If you see such a product, I would advise you to avoid it, as this substance will prevent you from reaping the benefits of high cocoa percentage.

- **Coffee**

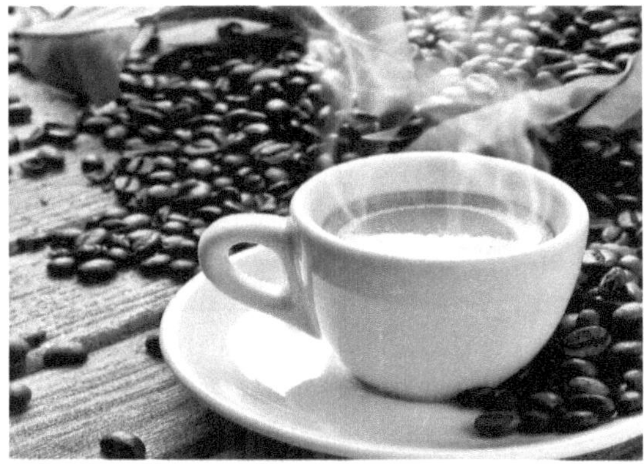

This is a drink enjoyed by most adults out there, and it is considered indispensable by most of them. We even believe that we can function without a cup of coffee to start within the morning. Obviously, that's not true, but we can honestly believe that coffee significantly improves our productivity and our daily activities. The caffeine acid is a nutrient known to activate sirtuins, so there's more to drinking coffee than a popular and a very pleasant social activity. Coffee houses all over the world are making serious money out of people's addiction to hanging out and drinking coffee. It is no secret that coffee is very good for your metabolism. It literally boosts your energy level, so you can even work out at full intensity. However, you don't want to drink too much coffee, as coffee excess can be harmful to your blood pressure. Most specialists would agree that 2 to 4 cups of coffee per day is the optimum daily quota. There are too many people who can't stand the taste of coffee and put a lot of sugar with it. Whether you use regular sugar, brown sugar, or even honey, I would rule them out. If you really want to sweeten your coffee, use stevia instead or drink the coffee in its pure form.

• Extra-Virgin Olive Oil

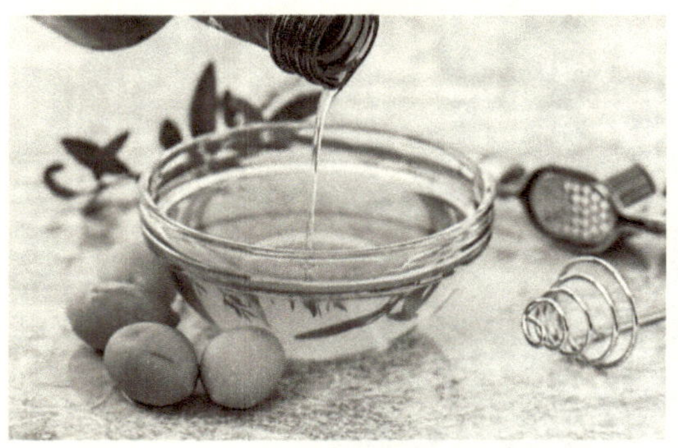

This oil is perhaps the healthiest form of fats you can think of, and it is not missing from any salad in the Mediterranean diet. The health benefits of consuming this oil are countless. It prevents and fights against diabetes, different types of cancer, osteoporosis, and many more. Plus, the extra-virgin olive oil can be associated with increased longevity, as it also has anti-aging effects. You can easily find this type of oil in most supermarkets, so you don't have any excuse to exclude it from your sirtfood diet. This oil has the right nutrients to activate the sirtuin gene in your body.

• Garlic

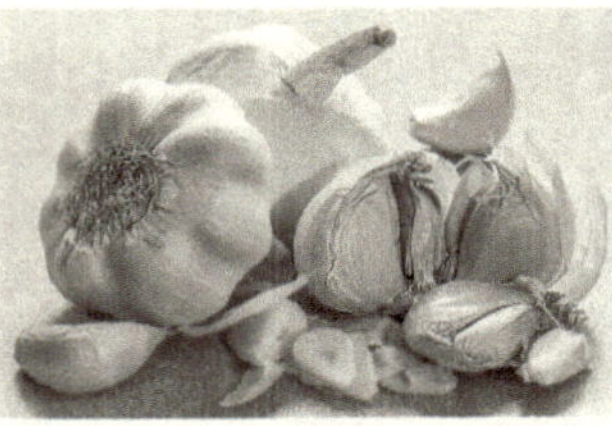

As you probably know, it has an antifungal and antibiotic effect and has been successfully used to treat stomach ulcers. Plus, it can be used to remove waste products from your body. It has amazing effects on your blood pressure, blood sugar level, and your heart. So why refuse this delicious food to feel healthy? Garlic contains allicin, a nutrient capable of triggering sirtuins, but this nutrient can only be valued if the garlic clove is crushed. Therefore, if you want to reap the benefits of this food, you have to avoid cooking it immediately. You need to crush it first and let the allicin form (should take around 10 minutes) before cooking it. This is the right way to use garlic in a sirtfood diet.

• Green Tea

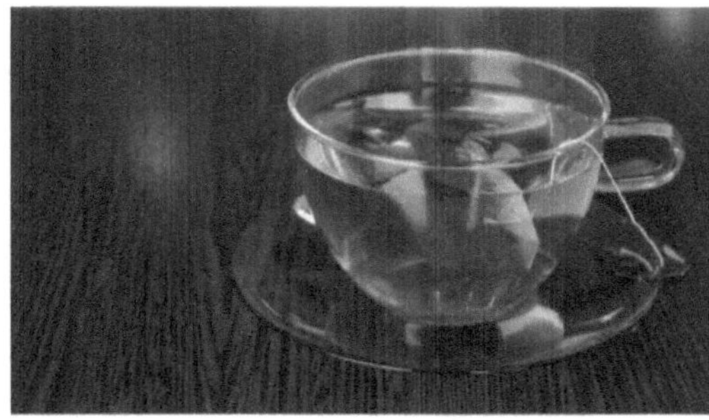

In some cultures, drinking tea is as popular as drinking coffee, but what if you find the tea assortment that works best for you? It is true that you can have tea from various medicinal plants, and they all have positive effects on your health. However, most of these plants are focused on preventing or fighting a specific disease.

Have you ever thought about drinking tea for your well-being or to feel great? Well, this is what green tea is for. First appeared in Asia, green tea has become very popular in Western culture. It has plenty of antioxidants. It can be used for detox, and it speeds up your metabolism. But there's a lot more to drinking green tea than these. Its benefits expand to preventing and fighting against diabetes, heart diseases, and cancer in incipient forms. When it comes to sirtuins activation, green tea contains EGCG (epigallocatechin), which is known to be a very powerful sirtuin activator. Well, this is what normal green tea can do for you, but if you want more obvious results, then you need to go for the matcha tea, which is the super green tea. This form of green tea is powdered, and it gets dissolved directly in the water, unlike normal green tea, which is prepared through an infusion. Therefore, this method of preparation allows the tea to have seriously increased levels of EGCG, in comparison with other forms of green tea. It is no wonder why Zen priests consider matcha as the ultimate medical and mental remedy.

• Kale

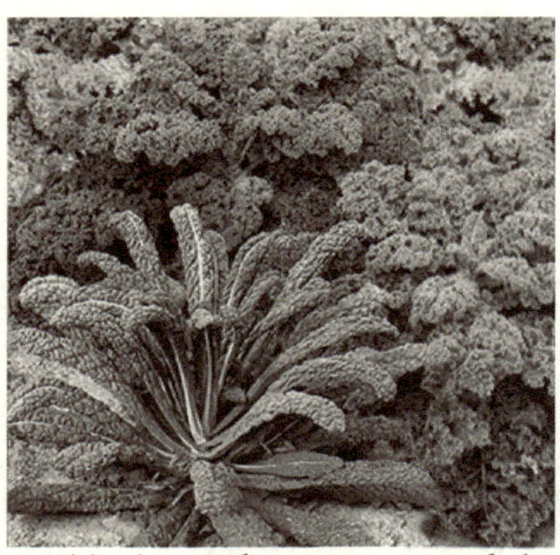

You can never go wrong with some leafy greens, and this is applicable for kale as well. Perhaps not many of you have tried it before, but it is totally worth it. Over the last few years, kale has gained a lot of popularity and appreciation from both nutritionists and consumers, and they have all the reasons to like and appreciate it. But what's all the fuss about it? How come this vegetable has become so popular lately? We can go on for hours talking about the health benefits of kale, but let's stick to the ones relevant to sirtuins, shall we? This leafy green is one of the best sources of kaempferol and quercetin, nutrients capable of triggering sirtuins. Therefore, kale should not be missing from your sirtfood diet, and you can easily make your own juices using it. Another great fact about kale is that it is not something exotic, a very rare vegetable available on a remote tropical island. This leafy green can be grown locally, so it is very accessible and affordable.

• Medjool Dates

If you have the chance to go to any country of the Middle East or the Arabian Peninsula, you will find that dates are a very common snack. Dehydrated, covered in chocolate, or in a fresher form, dates are perhaps the most common snack you can find over there. Now you are probably wondering if it has any health benefits, especially if you find out that Medjool dates have around 66 percent sugar. But sugar in this form is a lot less harmful than processed or refined sugar, which doesn't have any sirtuin-activating properties and can be easily linked to weight gain (even obesity), heart disease, and diabetes.

This is something to think of, a true dilemma. How come a fruit with 66 percent natural sugar can have any positive effects on your health? As it turns out, Medjool dates (consumed moderately) don't have noticeable effects when it comes to raising the blood sugar level. In fact, they have opposite effects, as moderate consumption can lead to lower heart disease or diabetes risk. In recent years, these fruits have become very interesting for nutritionists and for medical researchers in general, as they are seen as a potential cure for different diseases. This is the beauty of the sirtfood diet. It allows you to indulge in sweet treats without feeling guilty. But remember, moderate consumption only! You don't have to eat large quantities of Medjool dates.

- ## Parsley

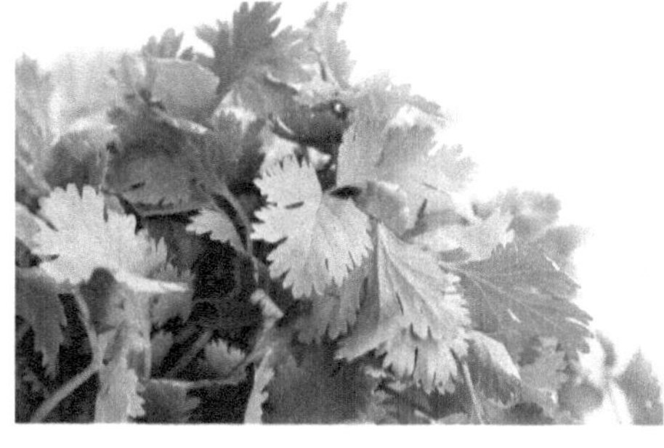

The parsley leaves are extremely frequent in recipes, so it is not missing from the sirtfood diet. You can chop them and toss them in your meal or use a sprig for decorative purposes. But parsley is not for decorating your plate, as you are not trying to impress a jury of famous chefs. This is an underrated plant. In ancient times, parsley was eaten after a meal to refresh the breath, so it was not considered as part of a meal. The sirtfood diet puts parsley where it belongs, and that is on your plate as an important part of your meal. With its refreshing and vibrant taste, parsley finally receives the respect it deserves.

If you are wondering what's so special about it, keep in mind that parsley is a great source of apigenin, which is (you guessed it) a sirtuin-activating nutrient. This nutrient can rarely be found in such quantities in other foods. This is why parsley is so special. Apigenin is good for activating sirtuins, as it can help you relax and easily fall asleep (by connecting with the benzodiazepine receptors in your brain). Therefore, head to the closest supermarket or grocery store to buy fresh parsley for your meals.

- **Red Endive**

This vegetable is one of the latest discoveries in the world of plants. How come? It was discovered by accident in 1830 when a Belgian farmer who stored chicory roots in his cellar, forgot about them, and discovered them with white leaves that happened to be crunchy, tender, and delicious. The recently found plant is growing all over the world and plays a major role in a sirtfood diet because of its high concentration of luteolin, a sirtuin-activating nutrient. On top of that, luteolin has been used to improve sociability for autistic children. Judging by the way most of us raise our kids (isolated, just with technology), more and more kids tend to be autistic. Therefore, the red endive can be very helpful in this case, so you better include it on your shopping list.

This veggie can have a crisp texture. At first bite, you will feel a sweet flavor, but that sweetness is followed by a mild bitterness. A great way to raise the quantity of luteolin in your diet is to add red endive to your salad. Naturally, pour some extra-virgin olive oil to make it more sirtuin-activating. Endives can come in different colors. It would be great if you can find them red (as these are the best), but you can settle for yellow ones as well.

- **Red Onions**

If you are only eating onions as O-rings with your burger, then you better rethink the way you consume this incredible vegetable. This type of onion has a sweeter taste (compared to yellow onion). It has plenty of antioxidants, and it is known to fight against inflammation, heart diseases, and diabetes. But there's a lot more to the red onion than meets the eye. It is a great source for quercetin, an amazing sirtuin-activating nutrient that is believed to enhance sports performance. Therefore, the red onion is a must in your sirtfood diet.

• Red Wine

The Mediterranean diet encourages the consumption of red wine, and there are plenty of reasons why you should consider the moderate consumption of it. We are not going to talk about the effects it has over your blood, blood sugar level, and so on. Not even about how moderate consumption can decrease the death rates by heart disease. Or about how red wine can prevent common colds and cavities (yes, it can even improve your oral health). Red wines like Merlot, Cabernet Sauvignon, or Pinot Noir have an incredible concentration of polyphenol to activate your sirtuins. Again, moderate consumption is essential, so one glass of wine should be more than enough.

• Soy

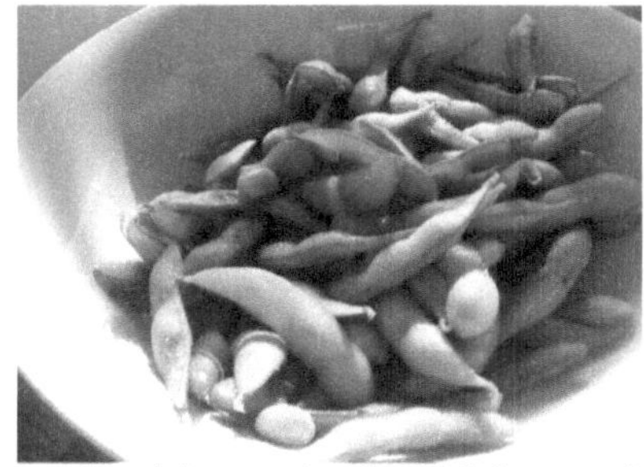

There is a whole food-processing industry behind soy, as it is used to create food products for vegetarians. But let's face it, drinking soy milk will not activate your sirtuins. Industrially processed food is not very recommended for your health, so it should be excluded from your sirtfood diet. In natural form, soy contains formononetin and daidzein, two great sirtuin-activating nutrients. For this kind of diet, you need to consider soy in different forms. Consider tofu (the vegan protein boost), or different fermented forms of soy, such as natto, tempeh, or miso (a Japanese fermented paste with an intense umami flavor).

- ## Strawberries

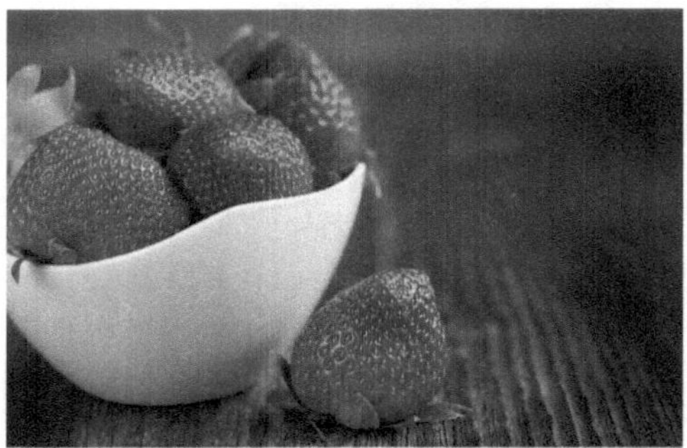

Of all the fruits out there, strawberries are among the ones with the most health benefits. Yes, they are sweet, but they happen to have a very high concentration of fisetin, a nutrient that can activate sirtuins. What is very confusing is that strawberries are known to prevent heart diseases, diabetes, cancer, osteoporosis, and Alzheimer's disease. They are even associated with healthy aging. Although they are sweet, 3½ ounces of strawberries only contain a teaspoon of sugar.

The consumption of this fruit can lower the insulin demand, basically turning the food into a sustainable energy releaser. There is research claiming that eating strawberries has similar effects on drug therapy for a person suffering from diabetes.

- ## Turmeric

You are probably familiar with the effects ginger has on your overall health, but you don't know what turmeric can do for you. This plant is related to ginger, and it is very appreciated throughout Asia for medical and culinary reasons. India is responsible for 80 percent of the whole turmeric on the planet, and some nutritionists refer to it as the "golden spice" or "India's gold." Why is that? Because it contains curcumin, a very rare sirtuin-activating nutrient. Unfortunately, this nutrient is very poorly assimilated when eaten, but if you cook it in liquid, add some fat and black pepper, you can boost its absorption. It is no wonder that turmeric fits so well in traditional Indian cuisine, as it goes very well with black pepper and ghee in hot dishes or curries.

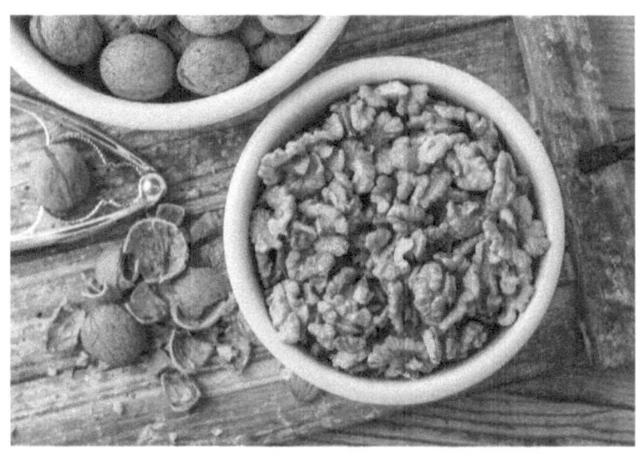

• Walnuts

As it happens, the walnut tree is the oldest food tree known to humans, as it was discovered around 7,000 BCE. Its original location was in ancient Persia (modern-day Iran), and now this tree is spread all around the world, as it can easily adapt to different climates of the globe. In the United States, walnuts are a success story. California is the biggest producer of walnuts in the United States, responsible for 99 percent of the US commercial supply and for three-quarters of the walnut trade worldwide. Without any doubt, walnuts are the best nuts when it comes to health. They may have a higher concentration of fats (healthy fats though) and more calories compared to other fruits, but the consumption of walnuts is associated with lowering the risk of diabetes, preventing cardiovascular diseases, and decreasing body weight. Walnuts are also known for their anti-aging effects, and to make you even more "nuts" about walnuts, their nutrients are known to activate sirtuins.

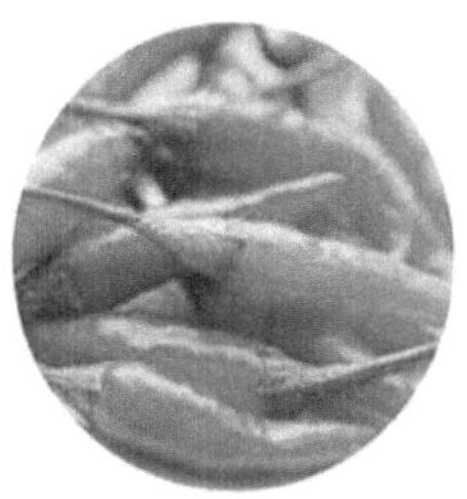
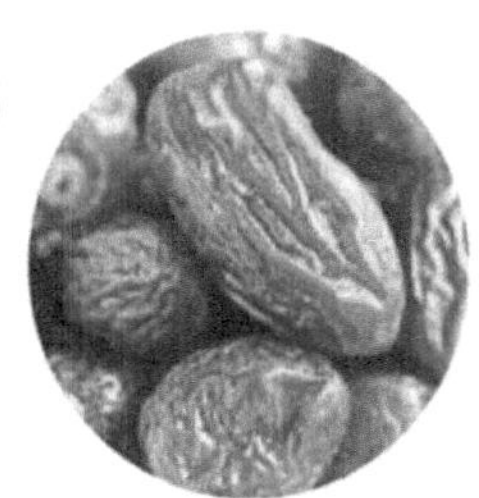

TOP 20 SIRTFOODS

Bird's-eye chilli
Buckwheat
Capers
Celery
Cocoa
Coffee
Extra virgin olive oil
Green tea (especially
matcha green tea)
Kale
Lovage
Medjool dates
Parsley
Red chicory
Red onion
Red wine
Rocket
Soy
Strawberries
Turmeric
Walnuts

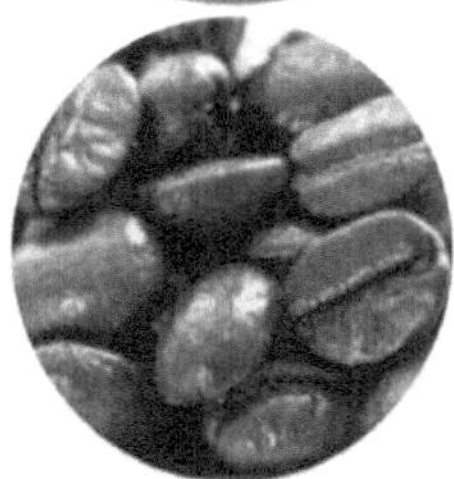
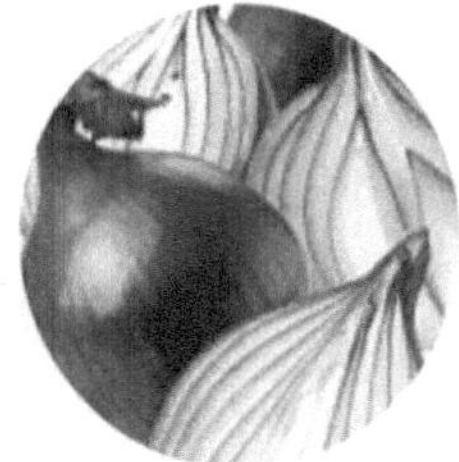
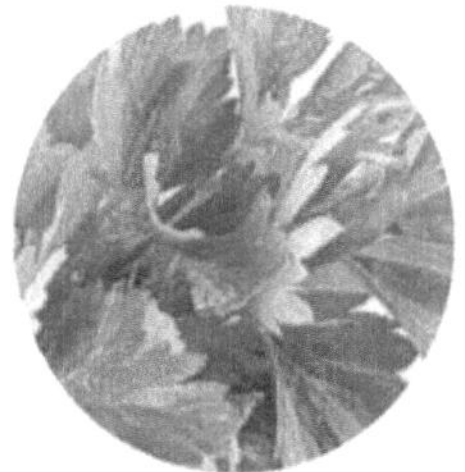
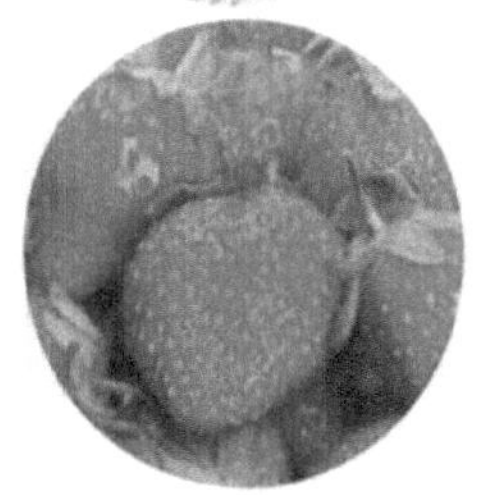

Raw honey	Spelt flour	Tofu
Buckwheat	Buckwheat flour	Onions
Almond milk	Baking powder	Garlic cloves
Ground cinnamon	Salt	Curry powder
Vanilla extract	Olive oil	Mushrooms
Blueberries	Coconut sugar	Carrots
Medjool dates, pitted	Smith apples	Cannellini beans
Cacao powder	Kale	Tomatoes
Flaxseed	Coconut oil	Eggs
Almond butter	Salmon	Soy sauce
Ice cubes	Chia seeds	Blackcurrants
Lime	Ginger	Celery
Basil leaves	Vegetable broth	Chicory (red)
Arugula	Sugar	Lovage
Strawberries	Broccoli florets	Citrus fruits- oranges, grapefruits
Parsley	Capers	Medjool dates
Turmeric	Cocoa	Fish oil
Green tea	Coffee	Red wine

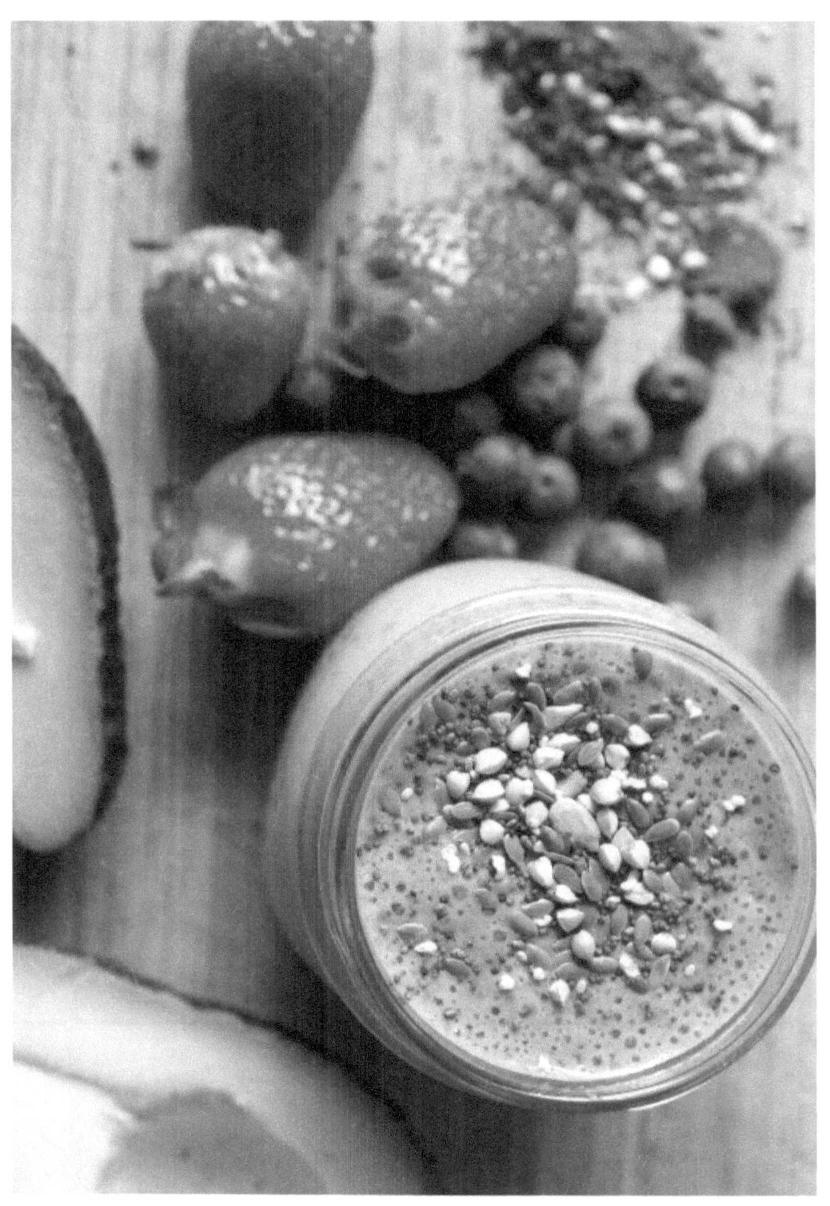

Phase 1 day 1, 2,3

Day 1:

Breakfast: Buckwheat Porridge

Lunch: Lentils & Greens Soup

Dinner: Apple Pancakes

Day 2:

Breakfast: Buckwheat Pancakes

Lunch: Salmon & Kale Scramble

Dinner: Chocolate Waffles

Day 3:

Breakfast: Eggs with Kale

Lunch: Tofu & Veggies Curr

Dinner: Buckwheat Granola

Phase 2 day 4, 5,6,7

Day 4:

Breakfast: Kale Scramble

Lunch: Mushroom & Kale Frittata

Dinner: Strawberry, Apple & Arugula Salad

Day 5:

Breakfast: Chocolaty Date Smoothie

Lunch: Grapes & Rocket Smoothie

Dinner: Matcha Pancakes

Day 6:

Breakfast: Buckwheat Porridge

Lunch: Buckwheat Burgers

Dinner: Buckwheat Pancakes

Day 7:

Breakfast: Blueberry & Kale Smoothie

Lunch: Beans & Kale Soup

Dinner: Salmon & Kale Scramble

Chapter 12: Maintenance

Once you've made it to the second stage you no longer have to count calories. Your reset week is over and now you simply have to maintain your new, more healthful habits. From this point forward, your meals should be celebrations of the food you are consuming.

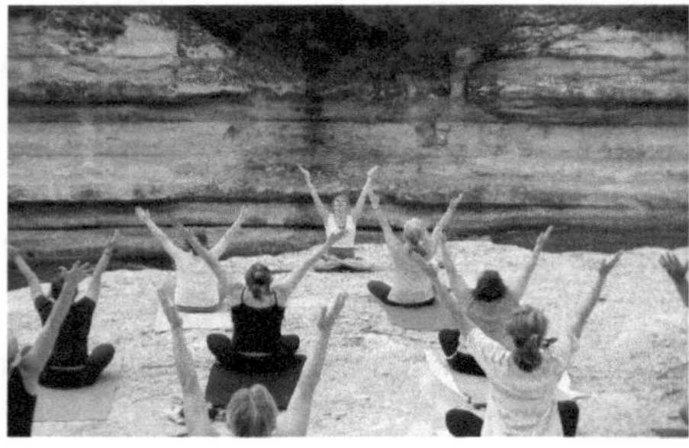

The goal of the Sirtfood Diet is to set you up for lifelong success incorporating these nutrient-dense sirtfoods into your daily life. The maintenance phase is a 2-week period to help you transition from your previous diet, beyond the dietary reset and into an eating routine that is founded on health.

During Stage 2, your commitment is going to be dedicated to finding a routine that fits nicely into your unique lifestyle. You want to create habits of health so that your daily food decisions become easier and more automatic over time, with sirtfoods being the natural solution to your hunger.

Even though you're no longer counting calories, there is a good chance you will continue to lose weight, if you have excess weight to lose. As long as you continue to enjoy plenty of sirtfoods in your life, your body will continue to find its health and natural, ideal weight. As your health improves, your body will better be able to communicate with you, sending you more stable hunger signals and telling you clearly when you are full.

During the next 2 weeks, you are encouraged to start your day refreshed with a green juice and then balance your metabolism smoothly with 3 full, sirtfood rich meals.

Nutrient Density

As you start to return you're eating habits back to a more consistent 3 meals per day, your primary focus should be on making sure that the majority of foods that make it to your plate are chosen for their nutritional content. Most important, their polyphenol content.

Stage 2 isn't about counting calories, but you should still be aware of how much you're feeding your body. Portion sizes have become drastically disproportionate to our health needs in recent years, so it may take a bit of experimentation to find your own, personal healthy balance.

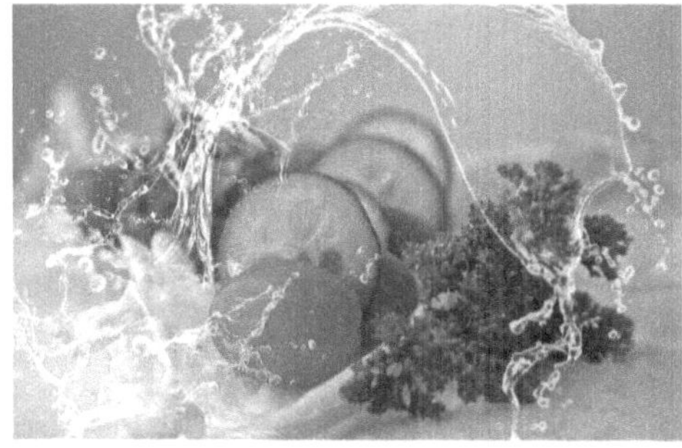

A really key component of healthy eating is setting time aside during your day to focus specifically on eating. Pay attention to your food instead of rushing to eat as quickly as possible before running out the door or eating mindlessly as you watch television. In both circumstances, you're not allowing your body to decide how much food it needs, which more often than not leads to over-eating. If instead, you sit down with friends or family, or even quietly by yourself, and pay attention to the process of eating, your body will give you cues when it's starting to fill up.

The Japanese have a mantra that they repeat before each meal: *hara hachi bu*. It's an ancient Confucian saying that reminds you to eat only until you're 80% full. This is very wise because it can take some time for your brain to realize your stomach is full. By the time you think you're full, you're probably already past this point.

As you learn how to listen to your biological hunger cues again, your taste buds will also be going through a natural adjustment period. They will need to re-learn what real, healthy food should taste like. You'll be surprised at how quickly your tastes will change, but as a general rule, you need to introduce a new few approximately 7 times before you will really learn to enjoy it. These next 2 weeks are designed to prove to you that, when you put your mind to it, you can learn to love healthy foods that are going to love your body in return.

Getting comfortable in your kitchen, if you're not already, is going to make a big difference in your life. We'll talk more about meal planning in a later chapter, but for now, it's a good idea to get familiar with some of the ingredients that are going to become staples in your home from now on. We talked about the versatility of buckwheat in the previous chapter and the value of matcha green tea.

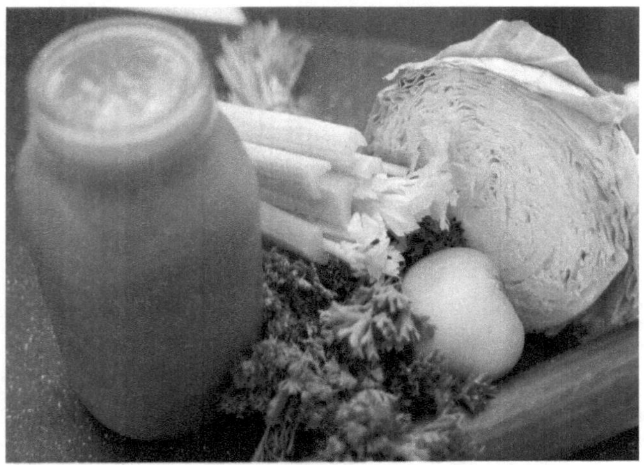

Two more ingredients that should be fairly easy to incorporate into a wide variety of meals, and easily find at almost any grocery store, are arugula, also known as rocket, and kale. For many years, spinach has been the leafy green to swap into your meals, but it's time to mix it up. Spinach is packed with nutrition and even polyphenols, but arugula and kale provide new flavors and textures for you to try, and also more variety in types of polyphenols. Just like you need a wide variety of vitamins, from A to K, so too will you be at your healthiest with a variety of polyphenols. So mix up your leafy greens, but always try to reach for the richest, darkest shades of green.

You can use greens in many different ways, so they're a highly versatile vegetable to always have in good supply in your fridge. You can, of course, add greens to your juice in the morning, and use them for the obvious salads and sandwich fillers. But great leafy vegetables are also delicious sautéed with a bit of olive oil and garlic or added to your buckwheat pasta dishes. Arugula has a spicy flavor and delicate leaves, whereas kale is woodier and brings a lot of texture to your dish, a good reminder to put your saliva to work as you chew your food well before swallowing. You can even sirtify your snack time; kale chips are a surprisingly simple treat to toast up in just a few minutes.

Focusing on adding more variety of leafy greens to your meals is a simple solution to increase the nutrient density of your food, but getting familiar with herbs and spices can bring even more variety to your meals.

Hot chili peppers, garlic, and parsley are probably all relatively familiar to you, but turmeric might not be as frequently used in your kitchen, though hopefully, it will be in your future.

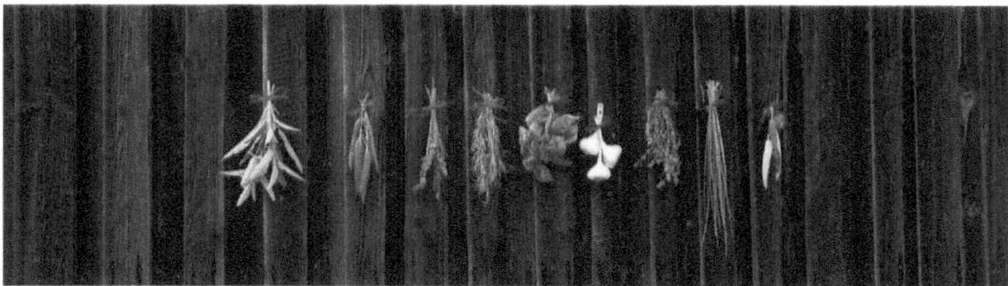

If you've ever enjoyed Indian food, you've most likely had turmeric. This spice is one of the most well-researched foods on earth, and it has been used in traditional medicines for thousands of years. Thanks to a phytochemical called curcumin, it is a natural anti-inflammatory agent that's very well known for its antioxidant capacity. It also happens to be very good at activating sirtuins.

Turmeric is widely used in Indian cuisine, responsible for the bright yellow hue of many curries, but it has a surprisingly mild flavor, making it suitable to add to a wide variety of dishes. Add a pop of color to your juices or smoothies, soups, stews, grain or pasta dishes, and it even makes a relaxing and delicious tea.

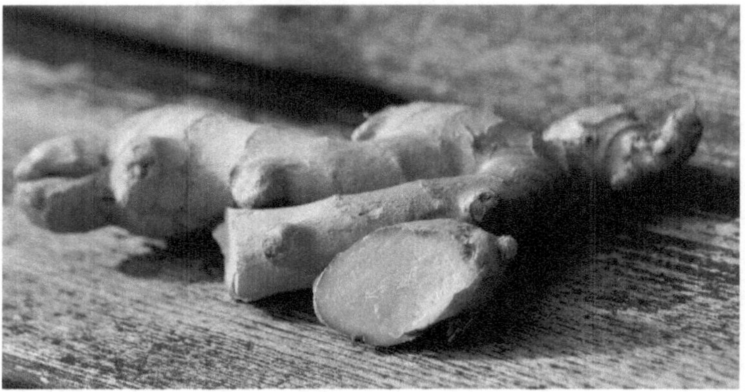

When you're planning your meals, it's important that you think beyond the focal ingredients and look for ways to add more sirtfoods, either as filler ingredients or even spices. Any extra sirtfood will increase the nutrient-density of your meals.

Digesting Sirtfoods

The more we learn about the health of our microbiome, or gut, the more obvious it is that it's a keystone to our overall health and enjoyment of life.

Many people are forced to plan their daily activities around the availability and accessibility of a toilet. This isn't a happy or comfortable situation to be in, but having a healthy digestive system can impact more than just your daily bowel movements, however distressing they may be. There is more and more evidence flooding the medical scene that shows how closely related our gut is to both our immune system and our brain health. Autoimmune disorders are on the rise, affecting millions of people in the USA alone. Bacterial infections that begin in your microbiome can directly affect learning and memory, and long-term intestinal damage can significantly increase your risk of cognitive decline.

When researchers looked very closely at the communication patterns between the gut and the brain, it turns out that only 10% of the messages start in the brain, usually during a stress response when the brain suggests the gut stops working temporarily so that energy can be put to better use elsewhere. In fact, if this happens and there is a lot of undigested food in waiting, your body may try to get rid of it quickly to save resources, and you could find yourself experiencing nervous vomiting or diarrhea in very stressful situations.

The other 90% of the communication, however, is traveling from our gut to our brain. This is logical, though it sometimes comes as a surprise to people. Your gut has more square footage that your entire skin does, so it is responsible for the intake of a lot of information about our nutritional status. It knows everything about what we are, or are not, feeding it in terms of nutrition. It's also responsible for training our entire immune system. If our brain needs information about our health, the first place it asks is our gut.

It makes sense then, that people who suffer from chronic digestive distress are going to be more at risk for diseases of the brain and mental health disorders.

The health of your gut depends on keeping a thriving community of healthy bacteria.

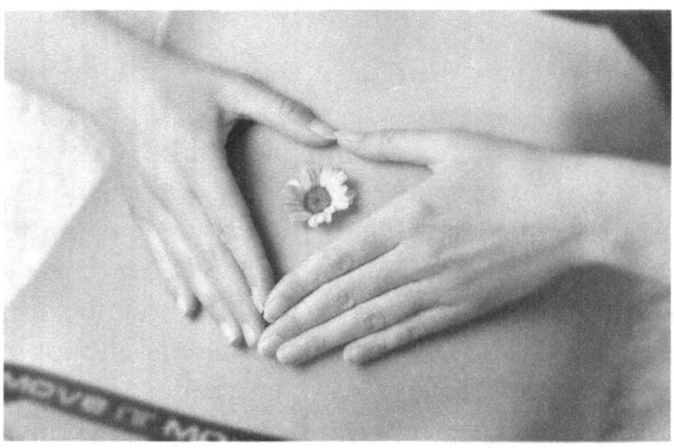

When you eat food, it gets digested in many stages, starting with your saliva and ending up in a mixture of highly acidic stomach juices. If this digestive process doesn't successfully break all the food particles down into their simplest components, you'll start to have trouble with the absorption of the nutrients from the food.

Sometimes, food particles that are only partially broken down will find their way into our bloodstream, where they can do damage and lead to an overactive autoimmune system. This is often called "leaky gut syndrome." Other times, we simply won't absorb the nutrition and we'll miss out on the value of the food we're eating.

To help make sure our food is properly digested, massive colonies of healthy bacteria line our entire digestive tract but primarily live in our intestines and colon. They feed on components of our food that we can't break down effectively, particularly fiber, which creates a symbiotic relationship between the bacteria and our gut.

Foods that feed these helpful bacteria are called prebiotics and primarily consist of specific kinds of fiber. Some common examples are garlic, onions and legumes or beans. Your body does not digest the fiber in these foods very well but they are enjoyed as the favorite nutrition source for the bacteria instead.

Certain types of food can also hurt and even kill the good bacteria in your microbiome. Flooding your gut with too much sugar and unhealthy fats will encourage the growth of harmful bacteria that, in time, can outnumber your good bacteria. Studies also show that some of the poisons that are used in conventional farming practices will not just kill the bugs that eat fresh produce, but it will also kill the bacteria in your gut.

Finally, antibiotics, though incredibly useful in killing harmful and potentially deadly bacterial infections, do not discriminate and will also kill healthy bacteria. If you ever need a course of antibiotics, one of the best things you can do for your long-term health is to follow this treatment with plenty of probiotic foods and possibly even supplements, to help repopulate your gut with good bacteria.

You may be wondering where these healthy bacteria come from in the first place though. They are introduced through specific foods as well: probiotics.

Probiotics are actually the live bacteria that colonize your gut and you consume them mainly through fermented foods, such as yogurt, sauerkraut and naturally picked vegetables, and fermented beverages like kombucha or kefir.

Sirtfoods are easily digestible, meaning that when the food reaches your stomach, it doesn't have a hard time breaking down the food to its nutritional components. This alone decreases the frequency of stomach upset, heartburn and other forms of digestive distress.

Additionally, nearly all plant-based foods are also high in fiber, which feeds the good bacteria and, in turn, reduces inflammation and therefore your risk factor for almost all diseases. Fiber is also one of the primary nutrients responsible for moving waste out of your body at an appropriate speed and consistency, reducing the experience of both constipation and diarrhea.

Even if we look beyond the value of sustaining healthy bacteria, sirtfoods are also very rich in polyphenols and other phytochemicals that have been found to improve digestion and neurodegenerative and cardiovascular diseases.

One great example is vitamin C. Most of the plant-based foods you find in this diet contain vitamin C, which helps our stomach regulate the production of hydrochloric acid and prevent bloating and acid reflux disorders.

As you can see, sirtfoods and the majority of edible plant-based foods, have many benefits for your body. However, because all people are unique, there are some circumstances in which adding copious amounts of sirtfoods to your diet quickly can be associated with some side effects.

For instance, the green juice and other fresh juices that make up an important part of the Sirtfood Diet are fermentable foods. This means they contain simple sugars and sugar alcohols that may irritate the stomach, sometimes causing gastrointestinal problems to people who suffer from issues like irritable bowel syndrome. If you currently experience regular digestive distress and, especially if you are taking any type of medication or treatment for issues with your gut, it is always a good idea to speak with your doctor about incorporating these foods safely.

You may not be able to drink the highly concentrated juices now, but after your gut has had some time to heal, you might be able to enjoy them later in your future.

On the whole, unless you have a specific sensitivity or allergy, incorporating plenty of sirtuin-activating foods into your daily meal routine will quickly improve the health of your digestive system

Fasting and Sirtfoods

Fasting has been researched by medical professionals to explore the wide range of benefits to health, including reducing risk factors for almost all diseases and decreasing the condition of aging. Much of the research done on sirtuins has discovered very similar health benefits.

Fasting and fasting-mimicking diets restrict or completely eliminate calorie consumption for a set period of time. During this time, your body is forced to access energy that is stored inside your cells in order to keep your body functioning. Most of us have a considerable amount of energy stored inside our fat cells, but when your metabolism is looking for a quick fix, it will take energy from anywhere it can find it, including your muscles and, more productively, repurposing damaged and dead cells that have accumulated inside your body.

A diet that centers around sirtfoods appears to achieve all the same results, without sacrificing any muscle mass in the process.

The reason for this overlap in beneficial factors is because fasting is a very effective way to activate sirtuins in response to the stress of having no incoming energy source. They are turned on as your body's natural defense against instant starvation. When you're following the Sirtfood Diet, however, our sirtuin genes are activated by the type of nutrition they are provided and then they change the way our body responds to all forms of stress. Instead of storing fat for a rainy day, they tell your cells to start burning fat instead, sending more energy to our muscles, reducing inflammation in our bodies and repairing damaged cells at the same time.

The results are very similar with the noticeable difference that, instead of potentially turning to our muscles and protein for energy as well as fat, as happens with fasting, activating our sirtuins actually protects and develops our muscles while burning fat. We're also accomplishing all of this while still providing our bodies with ample nutrition to heal and protect all the cells of our body and satiate our hunger and desire to eat.

A Sirtfood Diet also tends to be easier to follow and maintain in the long-term because it isn't asking you to live without food on a regular basis, and for the same reason, it can protect you more efficiently against malnourishment. Furthermore, restricting calories in any way can be dangerous and unsuitable for certain populations, which is why it is suggested that children under the age of 18, pregnant and breastfeeding women and anyone who is underweight or has a history of eating disorders skip Stage 1 of this diet. Fasting certainly would not be appropriate for these people, however, there is still a way for them to enjoy all the health benefits connected to fasting.

There's one more significant benefit of following a Sirtfood Diet to committing to a fasting protocol alone, and that is the quality of your nutrition. One of the reasons fasting has become so popular is because, during the feeding times, people are given free rein to eat anything they want, without any regard for quality and, depending on their goals, without even necessarily reducing the number of calories they normally consume. This can lead to very disordered eating and provides no assurances of nutritional support for your body.

Research has proven that the only way for your body to thrive and stay disease-free is to have consistent access to vitamins, minerals, fiber, antioxidants, and other phytonutrients. The Sirtfood Diet places these values at its core, making sure that you have everything you need to not just lose weight, but to heal your body naturally in the process and protect that health ferociously.

The Sirtfood Diet is designed to keep your body burning fat and protecting each individual cell in your body every day of the week, not simply charging into action for a few hours on the tail end of your fasted state, however frequent that may be.

Summary & Action Plan

When you're planning meals, it's important that you don't just eat the same foods you're used to eating and, if you do, at least improve them by adding a collection of sirtfoods to the dishes you're familiar with. For Stage 2 of the Sirtfood Diet it's best to eat primarily plant-based sirtfoods along with high-quality proteins and fats, but transitioning from a Standard American Diet can be a learning process. Have patience with yourself and be willing to experiment with new vegetables, spices, and even nuts, seeds and legumes. Variety truly is the spice of life.

Digestion is too often taken for granted, but it is a very complex process that seriously impacts our well-being and enjoyment of life. By following the Sirtfood Diet, you will be providing your gut with all the fiber, prebiotics and probiotics, as well as phytonutrition it needs to properly digest your food and keep your immune system thriving.

Stage 2 doesn't require you to count calories or restrict your calories in any way, but if you continue to eat mainly sirtfoods, you will be able to enjoy many of the advantages of a fast, but without any of the drawbacks. By activating our sirtuin genes through food, rather than fasting, the fat-storage processes still shut down, encouraging your body to burn rather than store fat, but without the negative side-effects of temporarily reducing nutrition or impacting muscle quality.

No Caloric Restriction

- Enjoy 1 sirtfood green juice, and

- 3 main meals

Similar to the first phase, you're welcome to consume non-caloric beverages such as water, black coffee, and green or herbal teas at any time. It is highly recommended that you completely remove high-sugar beverages from your life completely, however, as soda and energy drinks do much more harm to your body than good.

You can organize your meals throughout the day as they suit your lifestyle, but it is recommended that you drink your green juice in the morning to spark your metabolism into high gear for the rest of the day. To get the most of the potential benefits of fasting while on the Sirtfood Diet, try to eat your evening meal no later than 7 and then give yourself at least 12 hours of digestive rest before drinking your green juice.

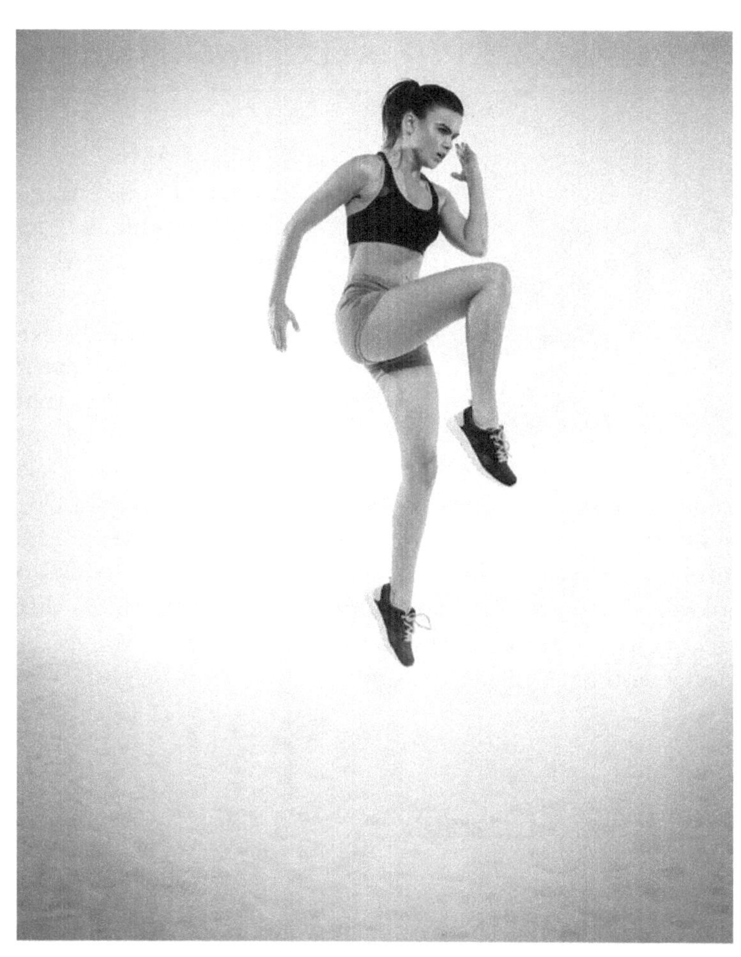

Chapter 13: Exercising and sirtfood diet

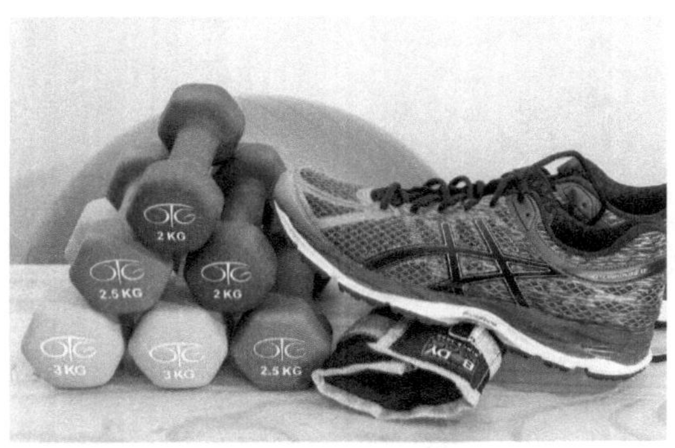

With 52% of Americans admitting that they think that its simpler to do their charges than to see how to eat steadily, it's fundamental to present a type of eating that turns into a lifestyle as opposed to a coincidental prevailing fashion diet. For a few of us it may not be that difficult to get thinner or hold a solid weight, however the Sirtfood diet can help the individuals who are battling. Be that as it may, shouldn't something be said about joining the Sirtfood diet with work out, is it fitting to stay away from practice totally or present it once you have begun the diet?

The Sirt Diet Principles

With an expected 650 million hefty grown-ups internationally, it's critical to discover smart dieting and exercise systems that are feasible, don't deny you of all that you appreciate, and don't expect you to practice all week. The Sirtfood diet does only that. The thought is that sure nourishments will dynamic the 'thin quality' pathways which are normally actuated by fasting and exercise. Fortunately certain nourishment and drink, including dull chocolate and red wine, contain synthetic substances called polyphenols that enact the qualities that copy the impacts of activity and fasting.

Exercise during the initial barely any weeks

During the main week or two of the diet where your calorie admission is diminished, it is reasonable to stop or lessen practice while your body adjusts to less calories. Tune in to your body and if you feel exhausted or have less vitality than expected, don't work out. Rather guarantee that you stay concentrated on the rules that apply to a solid lifestyle, for example, including satisfactory day by day levels of fiber, protein and products of the soil.

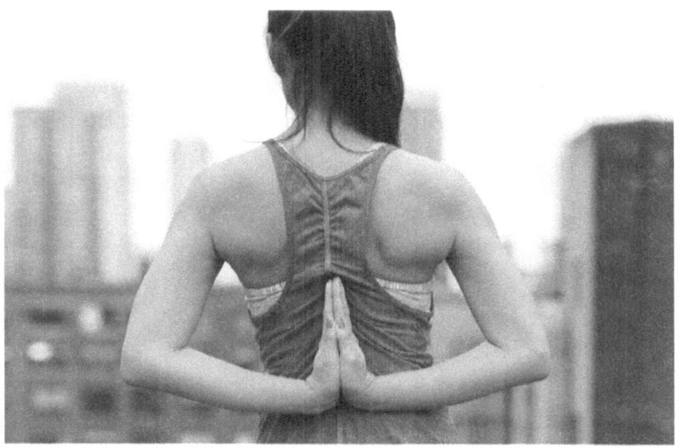

When you do practice it's critical to devour protein in a perfect world an hour after your workout. Protein fixes muscles after exercise, lessens irritation and can help recuperation. There are an assortment of plans which incorporate protein which will be ideal for post-practice utilization, for example, the sirt stew con carne or the turmeric chicken and kale serving of mixed greens. If you need something lighter you could attempt the sirt blueberry smoothie and include some protein powder for included advantage. The kind of wellness you do will be down to you, however workouts at home will permit you to pick when to work out, the sorts of activities that suit you and are short and helpful.

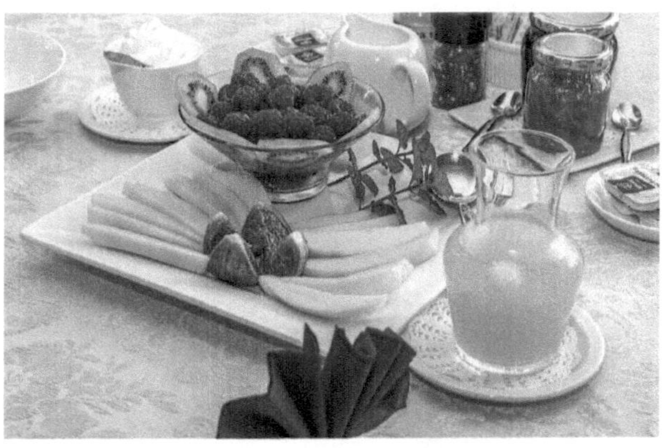

The Sirtfood diet is incredible approach to change your dietary patterns, shed pounds and feel more advantageous. The underlying not many weeks may challenge you yet it's imperative to check which nourishments are ideal to eat and which scrumptious plans suit you. Be benevolent to yourself in the initial barely any weeks while your body adjusts and take practice simple if you decide to do it by any stretch of the imagination. If you are as of now somebody who moderates or extreme exercise then it might be that you can carry on as ordinary, or deal with your wellness as per the adjustment in diet. Similarly as with any diet and exercise changes, it's about the individual and how far you can propel yourself.

Minerals and nutrients for which ladies may require supplements incorporate calcium, iron, Vitamins B6, B12 and D. Men, be that as it may, need to focus on fiber, magnesium, Vitamins B9, C and E. That reason applies to weight loss diets also. People's nourishment necessities sway which weight loss diets are increasingly compelling for each sex.

If you're similar to the vast majority, you've seen an astounding number of weight loss projects and patterns go back and forth; practically every one of them have their benefits and practically every one of them work incidentally. Weight the executives and therapeutic experts fight collectively that the deep rooted, proven blend of good sustenance and ordinary exercise is the most ideal approach to adequately shed pounds and keep it off

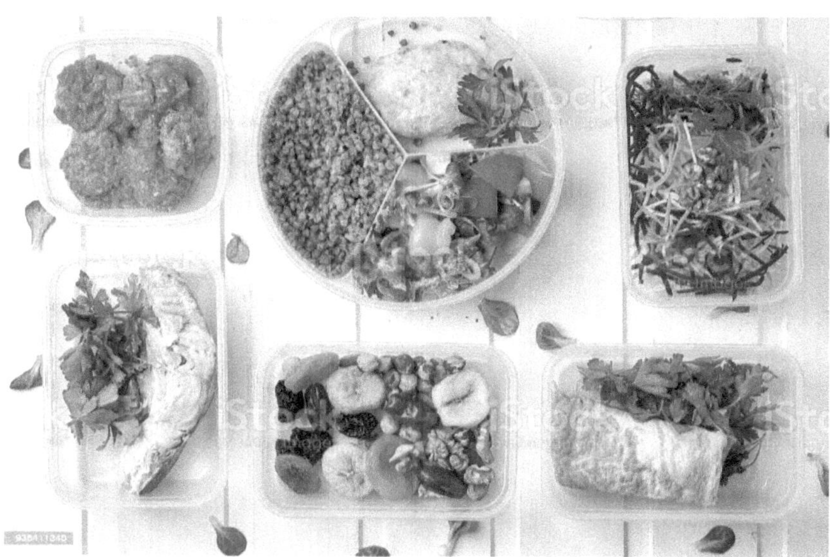

Chapter 14
Meal suggestion recipes

Buckwheat Porridge

Preparation time: 10 minutes Cooking time: 15 minutes Servings: 2

Ingredients

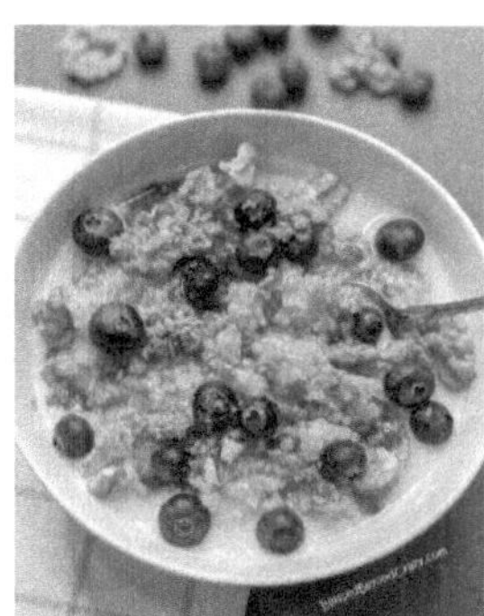

- 1 cup buckwheat, rinsed
- 1 cup unsweetened almond milk
- 1 cup water
- ½ teaspoon ground cinnamon
- ½ teaspoon vanilla extract
- 1–2 tablespoons raw honey
- ¼ cup fresh blueberries
-

Directions:

1. In a pan, add all the ingredients (except honey and blueberries) over medium-high heat and bring to a boil.

2. Now, reduce the heat to low and simmer, covered for about 10 minutes.

3. Stir in the honey and remove from the heat.

4. Set aside, covered, for about 5 minutes.

5. With a fork, fluff the mixture, and transfer into serving bowls.

6. Top with blueberries and serve.

Nutrition facts:

Calories 358 Fat 4.7 g Carbs 3.7 g Protein 12 g

Chocolaty Date Smoothie

Ingredients:

- 4-5 Medjool dates, pitted
- 2 tablespoons cacao powder
- 2 tablespoons flaxseed
- 1 tablespoon almond butter
- 1 teaspoon vanilla extract
- ¼ teaspoon ground cinnamon
- 1½ cups unsweetened almond milk
- 4 ice cubes

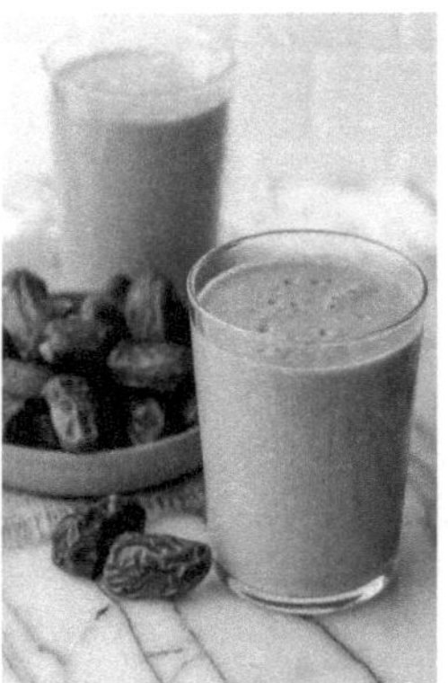

Directions:

1. Add all ingredients in a high-power blender and pulse until smooth.

2. Pour into two glasses and serve immediately.

Nutritional facts:

Calories 264 Fat 10.3 g Carbs 41.8 g   Protein 6.4 g

Matcha Berries Smoothie

Preparation Time: 10 minutes Servings: 2

Ingredients:

- 2 cups frozen mixed berries
- 2 Medjool dates, pitted
- ½ teaspoon fresh ginger, peeled and chopped
- 1 tablespoon chia seeds
- 2 cups unsweetened almond milk

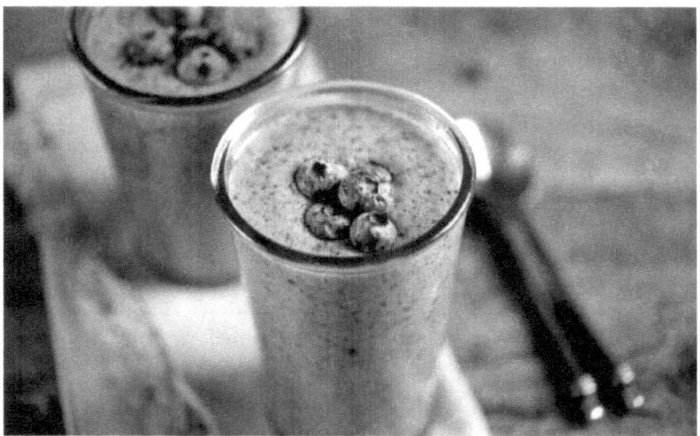

Directions:

1. Add all ingredients in a high-power blender and pulse until smooth.

2. Pour the smoothie into two glasses and serve immediately.

3.

Nutritional facts:

Calories 199   Fat 5.3 g   Carbs 37.3 g   Protein 3.6 g

Grapes & Rocket Smoothie

Preparation Time: 10 minutes Servings: 2

Ingredients:

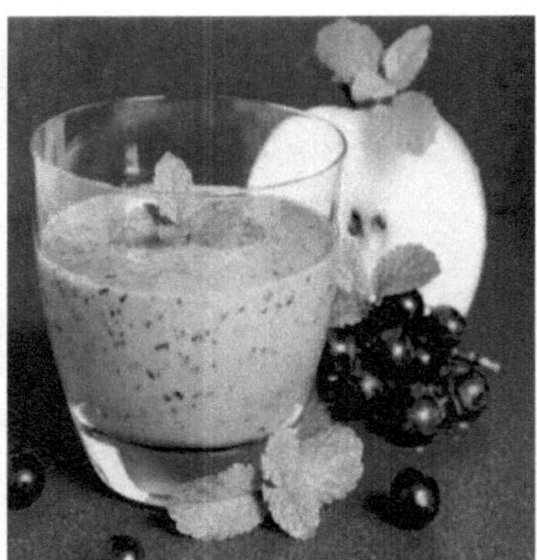

- 2 cups seedless green grapes
- 2 cups fresh rocket leaves
- 2 Medjool dates, pitted
- 1 teaspoon fresh lemon juice
- 1½ cups water
- 4 ice cubes

Directions:

1. Add all the ingredients in a high-power blender and pulse until creamy.

2. Pour the smoothie into two glasses and serve immediately.

Nutritional facts:

Calories 184 Fat 0.2 g Carbs 47.3 g Protein 1.3 g

Buckwheat Granola

Prep.Time: 15 minutes Cooking Time: 30 minutes Servings: 10

Ingredients:

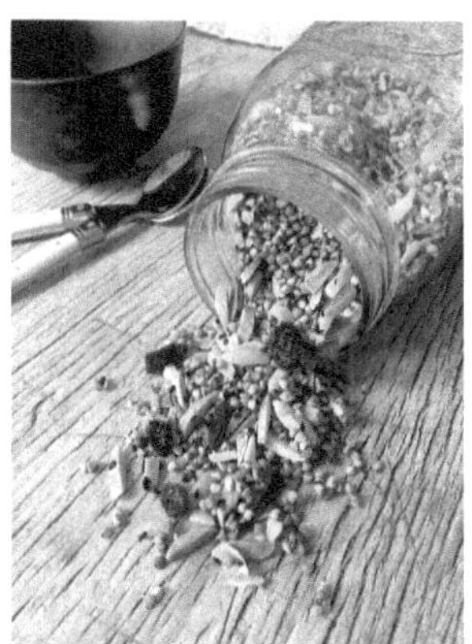

- 2 cups raw buckwheat groats
- ¾ cup pumpkin seeds
- ¾ cup almonds, chopped
- 1 cup unsweetened coconut flakes
- 1 teaspoon ground cinnamon
- 1 teaspoon ground ginger
- 1 ripe banana, peeled
- 2 tablespoons maple syrup
- 2 tablespoons olive oil

Directions:

1. Preheat your oven to 350 °F.
2. In a bowl, place the buckwheat groats, coconut flakes pumpkin seeds, almonds and spices and mix well.
3. In another bowl, add the banana and with a fork, mash well.
4. Add to the buckwheat mixture, maple syrup and oil and mix until well combined.
5. Transfer the mixture onto the prepared baking sheet and spread in an even layer.
6. Bake for approximately 25-30 minutes, stirring once halfway through.
7. Remove the baking sheet from oven and set aside to cool.

Nutritional facts:

Calories 252 Fat 14.3 g Carbs 27.6 g Protein 7.6 g

Matcha Pancakes

Prep Time: 15 minutes Cooking Time: 24 minutes Servings: 6

Ingredients:

- 2 tablespoons flax meal
- 5 tablespoons warm water
- 1 cup spelt flour
- 1 cup buckwheat flour
- 1 tablespoon matcha powder
- 1 tablespoon baking powder
- Pinch of salt
- ¾ cup unsweetened almond milk
- 1 tablespoon olive oil
- 1 teaspoon vanilla extract
- 1/3 cup raw honey

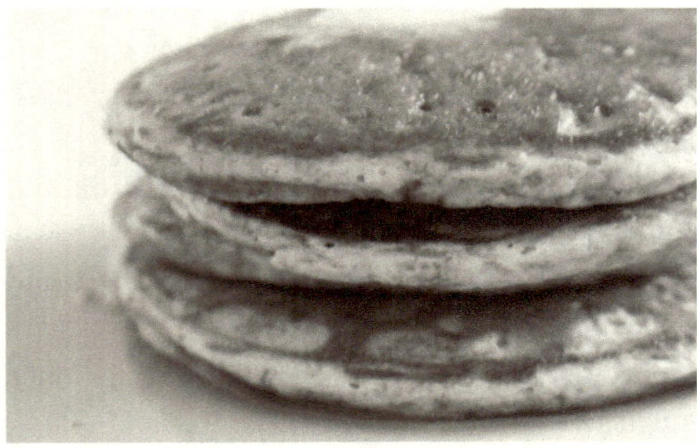

1. In a bowl, add the flax meal and warm water and mix well. Set aside for about 5 minutes.
2. In another bowl, place the flours, matcha powder, baking powder and salt and mix well.
3. In the bowl of flax meal mixture, place the almond milk, oil and vanilla extract and beat until well combined.
4. Now, place the flour mixture and mix until a smooth textured mixture is formed.
5. Heat a lightly greased non-stick wok over medium-high heat.
6. Add desired amount of mixture and with a spoon, spread into an even layer.
7. Cook for about 2-3 minutes.
8. Carefully, flip the side and cook for about1 minute.
9. Repeat with the remaining mixture.
10. Serve warm with the drizzling of honey.

Nutritional Facts:

Calories 232   Fat 4.6 g   Carbs 46.3 g   Protein 6 g

Apple Pancakes

Prep.Time: 15 minutes Cooking Time: 24 minutes Servings: 6

Ingredients:

- ½ cup buckwheat flour
- 2 tablespoons coconut sugar
- 1 teaspoon baking powder
- ½ teaspoon ground cinnamon
- 1/3 cup unsweetened almond milk
- 1 egg, beaten lightly
- 2 granny smith apples, peeled, cored and grated

Directions:

1. In a bowl, place the flour, coconut sugar and cinnamon and mix well.
2. In another bowl, place the almond milk and egg and beat until well combined.
3. Now, place the flour mixture and mix until well combined.
4. Fold in the grated apples.
5. Heat a lightly greased non-stick wok over medium-high heat.
6. Add desired amount of mixture and with a spoon, spread into an even layer.
7. Cook for 1-2 minutes on each side.
8. Repeat with the remaining mixture.
9. Serve warm with the drizzling of honey.

Nutritional facts:

Calories 93 Fat 2.1 g Carbs 22 g Protein 2.5 g

Salmon & Kale Scramble

Prep. Time: 3 minutes Cooking Time: 10 minutes Servings: 9

Ingredients:

- 2 cups fresh kale, tough ribs removed and chopped finely
- 1 tablespoon coconut oil
- Ground black pepper, as required
- ½ cup smoked salmon, crumbled
- 4 eggs, beaten

Directions:

1. In a wok, melt the coconut oil over high heat and cook the kale with black pepper for about 3-4 minutes.

2. Stir in the smoked salmon and immediately, reduce the heat to medium.

3. Add the eggs and cook for about 3-4 minutes, stirring frequently.

4. Serve immediately.

Nutritional facts:

Calories 257 Fat 17 g Carbs 7 gProtein 19.3 g

Mushroom & Kale Frittata

Prep. Time: 15 minutes Cooking Time: 30 minutes Servings: 5

Ingredients:

- 8 eggs
- ½ cup unsweetened almond milk
- Salt and ground black pepper, as required
- 1 tablespoon olive oil
- 1 onion, chopped
- 1 garlic clove, minced
- 1 cup fresh mushrooms, chopped
- 1½ cups fresh kale, tough ribs removed and chopped

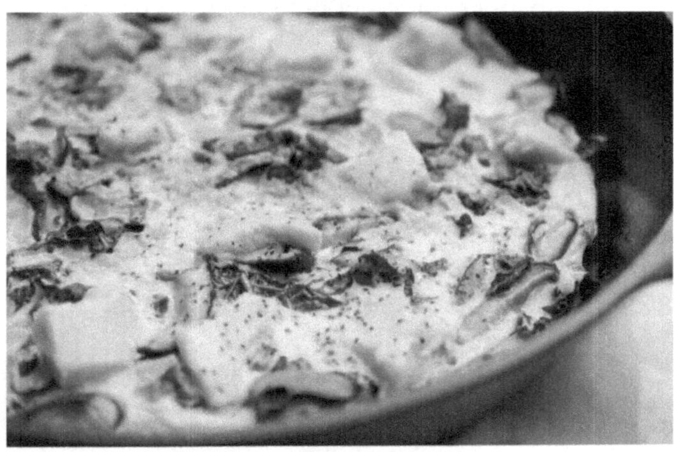

1. Preheat oven to 350 °F. .

2. In a large bowl, place the eggs, coconut milk, salt and black pepper and beat well. Set aside.

3. In a large ovenproof wok, heat the oil over medium heat and sauté the onion and garlic for about 3-4 minutes.

4. Stir in the mushrooms and cook for about 3-4 minutes.

5. Add the kale and cook for about 5 minutes.

6. Place the egg mixture on top evenly and cook for about 4 minutes, without stirring.

7. Transfer the wok in the oven and bake for approximately 12-15 minutes or until desired doneness.

8. Remove from the oven and place the frittata side for about 3-5 minutes before serving.

9. Cut into desired-sized wedges and serve.

Nutritional facts:

Calories 151 Fat 10.2 g. Carbs 5.6 g   Protein 10.3 g

Tofu, Kale & Mushroom Muffins

Prep. Time: 15 minutes Cooking Time: 30 minutes Servings: 6

Ingredients:

- 1 teaspoon olive oil
- 1½ cups fresh mushrooms, chopped
- 1 scallion, chopped
- 1 teaspoon garlic, minced
- 1 teaspoon fresh rosemary, minced
- Ground black pepper, to taste
- 1 (12.3-ounce) package lite firm silken tofu, pressed and drained
- ¼ cup unsweetened soy milk
- 2 tablespoons nutritional yeast
- 1 tablespoon arrowroot starch
- 1 teaspoon coconut oil, softened
- ¼ teaspoon ground turmeric

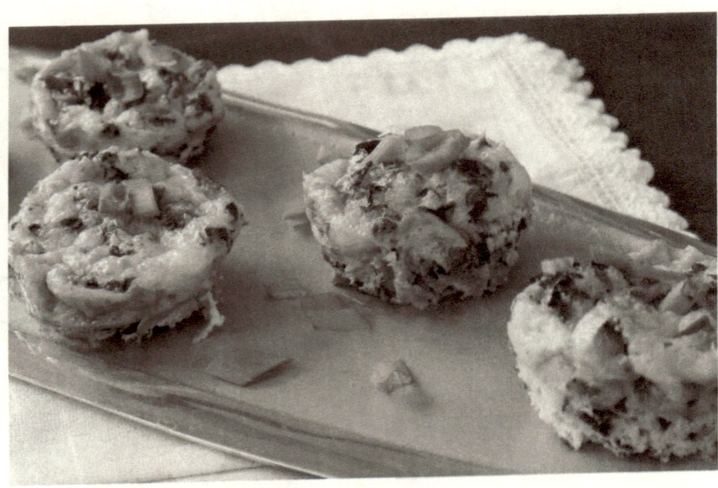

Directions:

1. Preheat oven to 375 °F.

2. Grease a 12 cups muffin tin.

3. In a non-stick skillet, heat the oil over medium heat and sauté the scallions and garlic for about 1 minute.

4. Add the mushrooms and sauté for about 5-7 minutes.

5. Stir in the rosemary and black pepper and remove from the heat. Set aside to cool slightly.

6. In a food processor, add the tofu and remaining ingredients and pulse until smooth.

7. Transfer the tofu mixture to a large bowl.

8. Fold in the mushroom mixture.

9. Transfer the mixture into the prepared muffin cups evenly.

10. Bake for approximately 20-22 minutes or until the tops become golden brown.

11. Remove the muffin pan from the oven and place it onto a wire rack for cooling for about 10 minutes.

12. Carefully, invert the muffins onto a platter and serve warm.

Nutritional facts:

Calories 82   Fat 4.4 g   Carbs 5.4 g   Protein 7.3 g

Blueberry & Kale Smoothie

Preparation Time: 10 minutes Servings: 2

Ingredients:

- 2 cups frozen blueberries
- 2 cups fresh kale leaves
- 2 Medjool dates, pitted
- 1 tablespoon chia seeds
- 2 teaspoons fresh ginger, chopped
- 1½ cups unsweetened almond milk

Directions:

1. Add all ingredients in a high-power blender and pulse until smooth.

2. Pour the smoothie into two glasses and serve immediately.

Nutritional facts:

Calories 230 Fat 4.5 g Carbs 48.8 g Protein 5.6 g

Strawberry & Beet Smoothie

Preparation Time: 10 minutes Servings: 2

Ingredients:

- 2 cups frozen strawberries, pitted and chopped
- 2/3 cup frozen beets, chopped
- 1 teaspoon fresh ginger, peeled and chopped
- 1 teaspoon fresh turmeric, peeled and grated
- ½ cup fresh orange juice
- 1 cup unsweetened almond milk

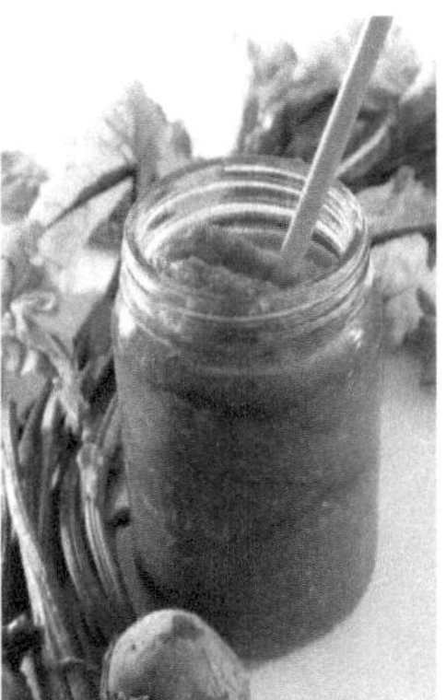

Directions:

1. Add all ingredients in a high-power blender and pulse until smooth.

2. Pour the smoothie into two glasses and serve immediately.

Nutritional facts:

Calories 130 Fat 2.1 g Carbs 27.5 g Protein 2 g

Beans & Kale Soup

Prep. Time: 15 minutes Cooking Time: 30 minutes Servings: 6

Ingredients:

- 2 tablespoons olive oil
- 2 onions, chopped
- 4 garlic cloves, minced
- 1 pound kale, tough ribs removed and chopped
- 2 (14-ounce) cannellini beans, drained
- 6 cups water
- Salt and black pepper, ground

Directions:

1. In a large pan, heat the oil over medium heat and sauté the onion and garlic for about 4-5 minutes.

2. Add the kale and cook for about 1-2 minutes.

3. Add beans, water, salt and black pepper and bring to a boil.

4. Cook, partially covered for about 15-20 minutes.

5. Serve hot.

Nutritional facts:

Calories 204 Fat 4.7 g Carbs 31.6 g Protein 11.5 g

Lentils & Greens Soup

Prep. Time: 15 minutes Cooking Time: 55 minutes Servings: 6

Ingredients:

- 1 tablespoon olive oil
- 2 carrots, peeled and chopped
- 2 celery stalks, chopped
- 1 medium red onion, chopped
- 3 garlic cloves, minced
- 1½ teaspoon ground cumin
- 1 teaspoon ground turmeric
- ¼ teaspoon red pepper flakes
- 1 (14½-ounce) can diced tomatoes
- 1 cup red lentils, rinsed
- 5½ cups water
- 2 cups fresh mustard greens, chopped
- Salt and ground black pepper, as required
- 2 tablespoons fresh lemon juice

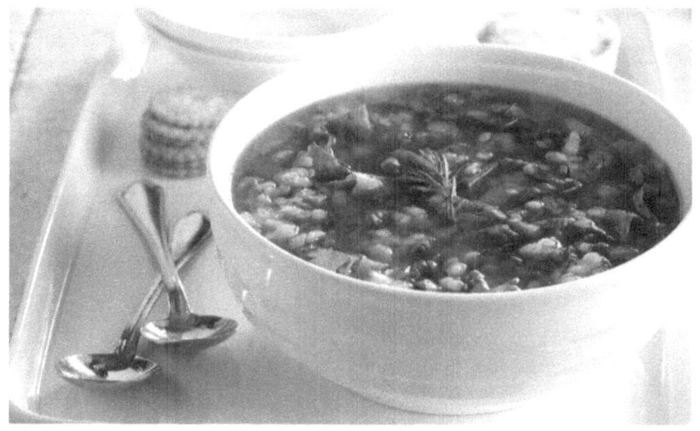

Directions:

1. Heat olive oil in a large pan over medium heat and sauté the carrots, celery and onion for about 5-6 minutes.

2. Add the garlic and spices and sauté for about 1 minute.

3. Add the tomatoes and cook for about 2-3 minutes.

4. Stir in the lentils and water and bring to a boil.

5. Now, reduce the heat to low and simmer, covered for about 35 minutes.

6. Stir in greens and cook for about 5 minutes.

7. Stir in salt, black pepper and lemon juice and remove from the heat.

8. Serve hot.

Nutritional facts:

Calories 174   Fat 3.1 g   Carbs 27.8 g   Protein 10 g

Tofu & Veggies Curry

Prep. Time: 20 minutes Cooking Time: 30 minutes Servings: 5

Ingredients:

- 1 (16-ounce) block firm tofu, drained, pressed and cut into ½-inch cubes
- 2 tablespoons coconut oil
- 1 medium yellow onion, chopped
- 1½ tablespoons fresh ginger, minced
- 2 garlic cloves, minced
- 1 tablespoon curry powder
- Salt and ground black pepper, as required
- 1 cup fresh mushrooms, sliced
- 1 cup carrots, peeled and sliced
- 1 (14-ounce) can unsweetened coconut milk
- ½ cup vegetable broth
- 2 teaspoons light brown sugar
- 10 ounces broccoli florets
- 1 tablespoon fresh lime juice
- ¼ cup fresh basil leaves, sliced thinly

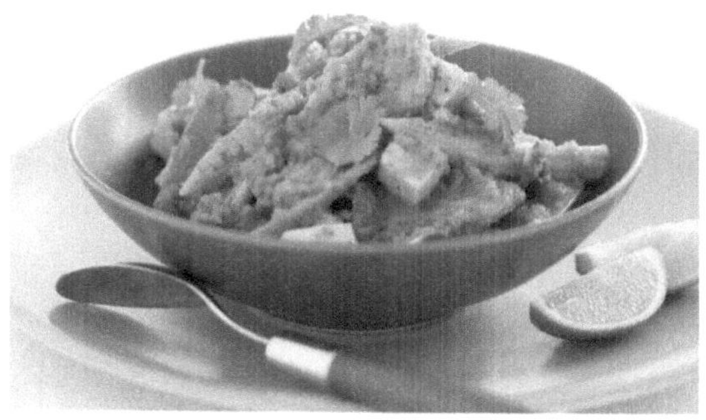

Directions:

1. In a Dutch oven, heat the oil over medium heat and sauté the onion, ginger and garlic for about 5 minutes.

2. Stir in the curry powder, salt and black pepper and cook for about 2 minutes, stirring occasionally.

3. Add the mushrooms and carrot and cook for about 4-5 minutes.

4. Stir in the coconut milk, broth and brown sugar and bring to a boil.

5. Add the tofu and broccoli and simmer for about 12-15 minutes, stirring occasionally.

6. Stir in the lime juice and remove from the heat.

7. Serve hot.

Nutritional facts:

Calories 184 Fat 11.1 g Carbs 14.3 g   Protein 10.5 g

Chocolate Waffles

Prep. Time: 15 minutes Cooking Time: 24 minutes Servings: 8

Ingredients:

- 2 cups unsweetened almond milk
- 1 tablespoon fresh lemon juice
- 1 cup buckwheat flour
- ½ cup cacao powder
- ¼ cup flaxseed meal
- 1 teaspoon baking soda
- 1 teaspoon baking powder
- ¼ teaspoons kosher salt
- 2 large eggs
- ½ cup coconut oil, melted
- ¼ cup dark brown sugar
- 2 teaspoons vanilla extract
- 2 ounces unsweetened dark chocolate, chopped roughly

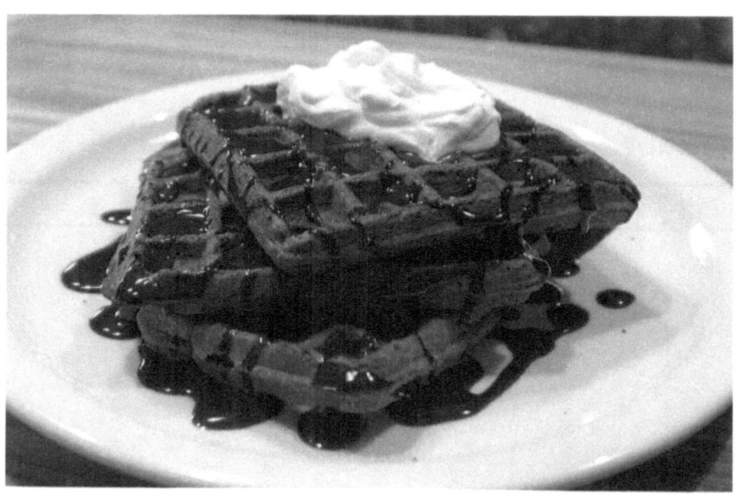

Directions:

1. In a bowl, add the almond milk and lemon juice and mix well.

2. Set aside for about 10 minutes.

3. In a bowl, place buckwheat flour, cacao powder, flaxseed meal, baking soda, baking powder and salt and mix well.

4. In the bowl of almond milk mixture, place the eggs, coconut oil, brown sugar and vanilla extract and beat until smooth.

5. Now, place the flour mixture and beat until smooth.

6. Gently, fold in the chocolate pieces.

7. Preheat the waffle iron and then grease it.

8. Place the desired amount of the mixture into the preheated waffle iron and cook for about 3 minutes or until golden brown.

9. Repeat with the remaining mixture.

10. Serve warm.

Nutritional facts:

Calories 295 Fat 22.1 g Carbs 1.5 g Protein 6.3 g

Buckwheat Pancakes

Prep. Time: 15 minutes Cooking Time: 15 minutes Servings: 5

Ingredients:

- 1 cup coconut milk
- 2 teaspoons apple cider vinegar
- 1 cup buckwheat flour
- 2 tablespoons ground flax seed
- 1 tablespoon baking powder
- ¼ teaspoon sea salt
- ¼ cup maple syrup
- 1 teaspoon extract, vanilla
- 1 tablespoon coconut oil

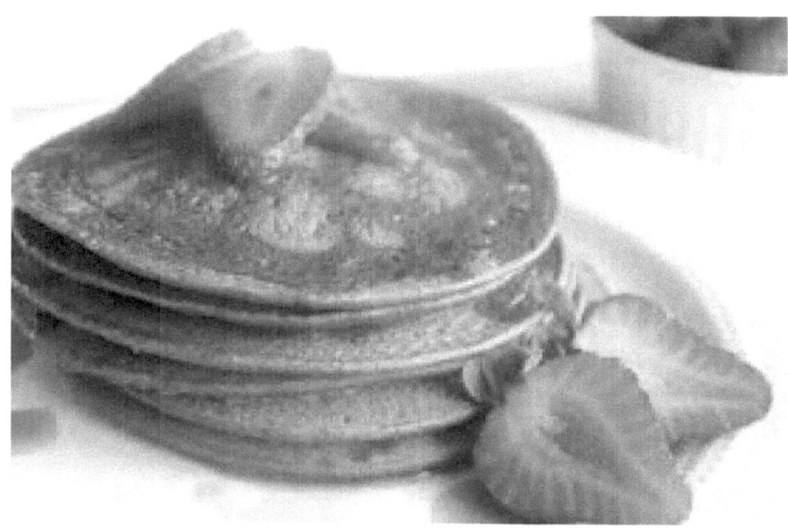

1. In a bowl, put together the coconut milk and vinegar. Set aside.

2. In a large bowl, mix together the flour, flax seed, baking powder, and salt.

3. Add the coconut milk mixture, maple syrup, and vanilla and beat until well combined.

4. In a nonstick skillet, melt coconut oil over medium heat.

5. Place about 1/3 cup of the mixture and spread in an even circle.

6. Cook for about 1-2 minutes.

7. Flip and cook for an additional 1 minute then remove from pan.

8. Repeat with the remaining mixture.

9. Serve warm.

Nutritional facts:

Calories 276 Fat 15.8 g Carbs 32.5 g Protein 4.7 g

Salmon & Kale Omelet

Prep. Time: 10 minutes Cooking Time: 7 minutes Servings: 4

Ingredients:

- 6 eggs
- 2 tablespoons unsweetened almond milk
- Salt and ground black pepper, as required
- 2 tablespoons olive oil
- 4 ounces smoked salmon, cut into bite-sized chunks
- 2 cup fresh kale, tough ribs removed and chopped finely
- 4 scallions, chopped finely

Directions:

1. In a bowl, place the eggs, coconut milk, salt and black pepper and beat well. Set aside.
2. In a nonstick wok, heat the oil over medium heat.
3. Place the egg mixture evenly and cook for about 30 seconds, without stirring.
4. Place the salmon kale and scallions on top of egg mixture evenly.
5. Now, adjust the heat to low and cook, covered for about 4-5 minutes or until omelet is done completely.
6. Uncover the wok and cook for about 1 minute.
7. Carefully, transfer the omelet onto a serving plate and serve.

Nutritional facts:

Calories 210 Fat 14.9 g Carbs 5.2 g Protein 14.8 g

Kale Scramble

Ingredients:

- 4 eggs
- 1/8 teaspoon ground turmeric
- Salt and ground black pepper, as required
- 1 tablespoon water
- 2 teaspoons olive oil
- 1 cup fresh kale, tough ribs removed and chopped

Directions:

1. In a bowl, place eggs, turmeric, salt, black pepper and water and with a whisk, beat until foamy.
2. In a wok, heat the oil over medium heat.
3. Stir in the egg mixture and immediately, reduce the heat to medium-low.
4. Cook for about 1-2 minutes, stirring frequently.
5. Stir in the kale and cook for about 3-4 minutes, stirring frequently.
6. Remove the wok from heat and serve immediately.

Nutritional facts:

Calories 183 Fat 13.4 g Carbs 4.3 g Protein 12.1 g

Eggs with Kale

Prep. Time: 15 minutes Cooking Time: 25 minutes Servings: 4

Ingredients:

- 2 tablespoons olive oil
- 1 red onion, chopped
- 2 garlic cloves, minced
- 1 cup tomatoes, chopped
- ½ pound fresh kale, tough ribs removed and chopped
- 1 teaspoon cumin, ground
- ¼ teaspoon red pepper flakes, crushed
- Salt and black pepper, ground
- 4 eggs
- 2 tablespoons fresh parsley, chopped

Directions:

1. Heat the oil in a big saucepan over heat and sauté the onion for about 4-5 minutes.
2. Add garlic and sauté for about 1 minute.
3. Add the tomatoes, spices, salt and black pepper and cook for about 2-3 minutes, stirring frequently.
4. Stir in the kale and cook for about 4-5 minutes.
5. Carefully, crack eggs on top of kale mixture.
6. With the lid, cover the wok and cook for about 10 minutes or until desired doneness of eggs.
7. Serve hot with the garnishing of parsley.

Nutritional facts:

Calories 175 Fat 11.7 g Carbs 11.5 g   Protein 8.2 g

Strawberry, Apple & Arugula Salad

Preparation Time: 15 minutes Servings: 4

Ingredients:

For Salad:

- 4 cups fresh baby arugula
- 2 apples, cored and sliced
- 1 cup fresh strawberries, hulled and sliced
- ¼ cup walnuts, chopped
- 4 tablespoons olive oil
- Salt and ground black pepper, as required

Directions:

1. For the salad, place all the ingredients in a large bowl and mix well.

2. For the dressing, place all the ingredients in a bowl and beat until well combined.

3. Pour the dressing over the salad and toss it all to coat well.

4. Serve immediately.

Nutritional facts:

Calories 243 Fat 19.1 g Carbs 19.7 g Protein 2.9 g

Buckwheat Burgers

Prep. Time: 20 minutes Cooking Time: 1¼ hours Servings: 4

Ingredients:

For Patties:

- ¾ cup dry buckwheat
- 1½ cups water
- Salt, as required
- 2 tablespoons olive oil, divided
- ½ of large red onion, chopped finely
- ½ of large carrot, peeled and grated
- ½ of celery stalk, chopped finely
- 1 fresh kale leaf, tough ribs removed and chopped finely
- 1 large cooked sweet potato, mashed
- 2 tablespoons almond butter
- 2 tablespoons low-sodium soy sauce

For Serving:

- 6 cups fresh baby kale
- 2 cups cherry tomatoes, halved

Directions:

1. Preheat your oven to 350°F.

2. Line a baking sheet with parchment paper.

3. For patties: heat a nonstick frying pan over medium heat and toast the buckwheat for about 5-6 minutes, stirring continuously.

4. Add the water and salt and bring to a boil over high heat.

5. Adjust the heat to low and cook, covered for about 15 minutes or until all the water is absorbed.

6. Meanwhile, heat 1 tablespoon of the oil in a skillet over medium heat and sauté the onion for about 4-5 minutes.

7. Add the carrot and celery and cook for about 5 minutes.

8. Stir in the remaining ingredients and remove from the heat.

9. Transfer the mixture into a bowl with buckwheat and stir to combine.

10. Set aside to cool completely.

11. Make 4 equal-sized patties from the mixture.

12. Arrange the patties onto the prepared baking sheet in a single layer and bake for about

13. Bake for approximately 20 minutes per side.

14. Divide the greens, tomatoes, cabbage and bell pepper onto serving plates.

15. Top each plate with 1 patty and serve

Nutritional facts:

Calories 340 Fat 12.9 g Carbs 51 g Protein 11.8 g

Conclusion

There are too many diseases and medical conditions caused by the food we eat. The quality of food has decreased dramatically over the past decades as the food-processing industry is now providing most of the food we consume. The more processed the food type is, the more harmful it is to your body. Food-processing companies are providing poison for the consumers, just to make more profits.

It is very difficult to find organic food nowadays as farmers use different chemicals to grow crops, fruits, and vegetables while animals are fed with concentrated food to grow very fast before being slaughtered for meat. All these chemicals are affecting the quality of food and our health.

There is way too much processed food introduced to us, and the Western way of life encourages the consumption of junk food. This is the main reason why diabetes and obesity are becoming very common in Western countries, especially in the United States.

This processed-food madness should now stop, and the sirtfood diet is here to do so. The logic behind this diet is very interesting, as it has a different approach to food than other diets. If you are struggling with your weight, don't have too much energy, and also have the suspicion of having different diseases caused by bad nutrition, then this is the diet for you. Don't hesitate and try the sirtfood diet now!

Did this book help you in some way? If so, I'd love to hear about it. Honest reviews help readers find the right book for their needs."

Weekly Meal Planner
Week of _________

	Breakfast	Lunch	Dinner
Mon			
Tue			
Wed			
Thu			
Fri			
Sat			
Sun			

Notes:

Weekly Meal Planner
Week of _________

	Breakfast	Lunch	Dinner
Mon			
Tue			
Wed			
Thu			
Fri			
Sat			
Sun			

Notes:

www.ingramcontent.com/pod-product-compliance
Lightning Source LLC
Chambersburg PA
CBHW031127250726
48655CB00002B/559